# CHALLENGES OF PSYCHOANALYSIS IN THE 21$^{ST}$ CENTURY

# CHALLENGES OF PSYCHOANALYSIS IN THE 21ST CENTURY

## Psychoanalysis, Health, and Psychosexuality in the Era of Virtual Reality

Edited by

José Guimón

*University of Geneva*
*Geneva, Switzerland*

and

Sara Zac de Filc

*President, Committee of Interregional Conferences*
*International Psychoanalytic Association*
*Buenos Aires, Argentina*

Kluwer Academic / Plenum Publishers
New York, Boston, Dordrecht, London, Moscow

Library of Congress Cataloging-in-Publication Data

Challenges of psychoanalysis in the 21st century: psychoanalysis, health, and psychosexuality in the era of virtual reality/edited by José Guimón and Sara Zac de Filc.

p. cm.

Includes bibliographical references and index.

ISBN 0-306-46677-5

1. Psychoanalysis—History—21st century—Congresses. 2. Internet—Psychological aspects. 3. Computer networks—Psychological aspects. I. Guimón, J. II. Zac de Filc, Sara.

BF172 .C435 2001
150.19′5′0112—dc21

2001038775

Proceedings of the International Conference on Challenges in Psychoanalysis in the 21st Century: Psychoanalysis, Health, and Psychosexuality in the Era of Virtual Reality, held September 15–17, 2000, in Geneva, Switzerland

ISBN 0-306-46677-5


233 Spring Street, New York, N.Y. 10013

http://www.wkap.nl/

10 9 8 7 6 5 4 3 2 1

A C.I.P. record for this book is available from the Library of Congress



Printed in the United States of America

# Preface

*Challenges of Psychoanalysis in the 21st Century*

Psychoanalysis has become a basic psychiatric science in very much the same way as the neurosciences or epidemiology. However, there is a certain present-day discrediting of psychoanalysis as a therapeutic tool stemming, to some extent, from the reluctance of psychoanalysts to submit their theories and practice to scientific scrutiny. Fortunately, there is a certain movement in psychoanalysis to introduce reliable measures that would allow for a scientific evaluation of its results as a therapeutic device.

Science is, like all human affairs, subject to the influences of changing fashions. Although there are great variations with respect to the role ascribed to psychotherapy in different countries, a certain upsurge of interest in psychoanalytic techniques is apparent nowadays even if it has resulted in a watered-down version of psychoanalysis called «dynamic psychiatry». In the United States, although fewer residents tend to initiate training in psychoanalytic institutes, a certain knowledge of dynamic principles and supervision of analytically-oriented psychotherapy is still included in most programmes. In Eastern European countries, a pedagogical and suggestive psychotherapy has prevailed but today dynamic psychiatry is gaining ground as seen in the widespread training in group analysis. In EC countries, psychoanalysis also seems to be holding its own. In the last three years a European Federation of Psychoanalytic Psychotherapy has been founded, including hundreds of psychiatrists in its three branches (child, group and individual psychoanalytic psychotherapy). A European Association of Psychotherapists has also appeared, uniting practitioners of all the known tendencies in psychotherapy. Psychoanalytic psychotherapy seems to be the strongest of these tendencies and psychiatrists are their most numerous and influential members.

This International Conference on Psychoanalysis and Virtual Reality was organised by the International Psychoanalytical Association and the Department of Psychiatry of the University of Geneva. We had in mind a series of concerns.

First, some of us thought that in the next century the differences between the conscious, unconscious and the pre-conscious will have to be reconsidered in view of the ever expanding concepts created by the advancement of Science and Technique. There will be virtual sexual acts over the Internet; ovum parthenogenesis will be possible without the intervention of the male, and clonic reproduction of the human being will be carried out in the laboratory. The child born in these circumstances will relate to a widening array of potential parental figures: the classical heterosexual couple, the single-parent family, the homosexual couple, the transsexual figure, etc. All this alters of course the classical Oedipal constellation and without doubt the gender identity of the child.

On the other hand we forecast that there will be attempts to undergo psychoanalytically oriented psychotherapy via the Internet in the same way that other kinds of psychotherapy are being «virtualized». But, should this happen, this will force us to re-define most psychoanalytical concepts and techniques.

Finally most of us believe that it is very likely that psychoanalysis as a psychotherapeutic tool will, in the $21^{st}$ Century, relate more to somatic, medical patients or to the 'worried well' than to psychiatric patients. These brief considerations on the scope of our deliberations in some way explain the diversity of the programme, but also probably justify its interest.

José Guimón
Sara Zac de Filc

# Contributors

**AISENSTEIN,** MARILIA Mme
*Member of Paris Psychoanalytical Society*
72, rue d'Assas
F - 75008 Paris
France
☎ 33 1 45 48 13 38
Fax 33 1 45 47 71 12
Email: mariliaais@hotmail.com

**CANESTRI,** JORGE Dr.
*Member of Italian Psychoanalytical Association*
Via Sesto Rufo 23
I - 00136 Rome
Italy
☎ 39 06 39 72 92 09
Fax 39 06 39 72 92 09
Email: canestri@mclink.it

**CRAMER,** BERTRAND Dr.
*Hon. Professor of Psychiatry, Member of Swiss Psychoanalytical Society*
10, Ch. Charles-Bonnet
1206 Genève
Switzerland
☎ 41 22 347 80 62
Fax 41 22 347 80 72
Email: bcramer@bluewin.ch

**EIZIRIK,** CLAUDIO LAKS Dr.
*Adjunct Professor of Psychiatry, Federal University of Rio Grande do Sul; Member of Porto Alegre Psychoanalytical Society*
783/307 Rua Marques do Pombal
BR - 90540-001 Porto Alegre, RS
Brazil
☎ 55 51 224 4364
Fax 55 51 224 4364
Email: ceizirik.ez@terra.com.br

**FLOURNOY,** OLIVIER Dr.
*Member of Swiss Psychoanalytical Society*
45, Avenue de Champel
1206 Genève
Switzerland
☎ 41 22 346 22 49
Fax 41 22 346 22 49
Email: flournoy@cosadgip.com

**FONAGY** PETER Professor
*Member of British Psycho-Analytical Society*
Sub-Department - Clinical Health Psychology
University College London, Gower Street
London WC1E 6BT
England, U.K.
☎ 44 20 7679 1943
Fax 44 20 7916 8502
Email: p.fonagy@ucl.ac.uk

**GITNACHT,** MAURICIO Dr.
*Member of Swiss Psychoanalytical Society*
13, Avenue Dumas
1206 Genève
Switzerland
☎ 41 22 346 23 07
Email: mauricio.gitnacht@span.ch

**GOLSE,** BERNARD Professor
*Professor of Psychiatry*
Psychiatre de l'Hopital St. Vincent de Paul
Service de Pédopsychiatrie
82, av. Denfert Rochereau

F - 75014 Paris
France
☎ 33 1 40 48 81 84
Fax 33 1 47 05 39 47
Email: b.golse@svp-ap-hop-paris.fr

**GUIMON,** JOSE Dr.
*Professor of Psychiatry, Member of Swiss Psychoanalytical Society*
Hôpital Belle-Idée
2, Ch. du Petit-Bel-Air
CH -1225 Chêne-Bourg
Switzerland
☎ 41 22 305 57 77
Fax 41 22 305 57 99
Email: jose.guimon@hcuge.ch

**HAYNAL**, ANDRE Dr.
*Hon. Professor of Psychiatry, Member of Swiss Psychoanalytical Society*
5, Boulevard des Philosophes
1205 Genève
Switzerland
☎ 41 22 781 06 00
Fax 41 22 348 19 56
Email: haynal@cmu.unige.ch

**HOUZEL,** DIDIER Professor
*Member of French Psychoanalytical Association*
Service de Psychiatrie de l'Enfant & de l'Adolescent
Centre Hospitalier Universitaire CLEMENCEAU
6, rue de l'Académie
F - 14000 CAEN
France
☎ 33 2 31 27 23 09
Fax 33 2 31 27 23 12
Email: houzel-d@chu-caen.fr

**MANZANO**, JUAN Professor
*Assoc. Professor of Child Psychiatry*
*President of Swiss Psychoanalytical Society*
Service médico-pédagogique
16-18, Boulevard Carl-Vogt
Case postale 50
1211 Genève 8

Switzerland
☎ 41 22 327 43 09
Fax 41 22 327 43 20
Email: juan.manzano@etat.ge.ch

**MARTINDALE,** BRIAN Dr.
*Associate Member of British Psychoanalytical Society*
31, Nassau Road, Barnes
London SW13 9QF
England, U.K.
☎ 44 20 8748 8795
Fax 44 20 8255 0181
Email: drbmartindale@cableinet.co.uk

**MICHELS,** ROBERT M.D.
*Walsh McDermott University Professor of Medicine*
*University Professor of Psychiatry*
*Member of American Psychoanalytical Association*
Cornell University - Medical College
418 East 71st Street - Suite 41
New-York NY 10021
USA
☎ 1 212 746 6001
Fax 1 212 746 3828
Email: rmichels@med.cornell.edu

**NICOLAIDIS,** NICOS Dr.
*Member of Swiss Psychoanalytical Society*
2, Ch. de la Tour-de-Champel
CH - 1206 Genève
Switzerland
☎ 41 22 347 13 54
Fax 41 22 346 47 87

**PALACIO-ESPASA,** FRANCISCO Professor
*Professor of Child Psychiatry, Member of Swiss Psychoanalytical Society*
Clinique de Psychiatrie Infantile
41, Chemin des Crêts de Champel
CH - 1206 Genève
Switzerland
☎ 41 22 346 55 80
Fax 41 22 789 28 47

**QUARTIER-FRINGS,** FLORENCE Dr.
*Member of Swiss Psychoanalytical Society*
40, Athénée
CH - 1206 Genève
Switzerland
☎ 41 22 347 74 77
Fax 41 22 347 74 77
Email: florence.quartier@worldcom.ch

**QUINODOZ**, JEAN-MICHEL Dr.
*Member of Swiss Psychoanalytical Society*
53A, Chemin des Fourches
CH - 1223 Cologny
Switzerland
☎ 41 22 349 49 42
Fax 41 22 349 49 42
Email: jmquinodoz@compuserve.com

**SCHTEINGART-GITNACHT,** ALICIA Dr.
*Member of Swiss Psychoanalytical Society*
22, Chemin de Roday
CH - 1256 Troinex, Geneva
Switzerland
☎ 41 22 784 32 33
Fax 41 22 346 23 07
Email: alicia.schteingart@span.ch

**TARGET**, Mary Dr.
*Member of British Psycho-Analytical Society*
Sub-Department - Clinical Health Psychology
University College London, Gower Street
London WC1E 6BT
England, U.K.
☎ 44 20 7679 1899
Fax 44 20 7916 8502
Email: m.target@ucl.ac.uk

**TIZON,** JORGE L. Dr.
*Member of Spanish Psychoanalytical Society*
Roger de Lluria 115
S - 08037 Barcelona
Spain

☎ 34 93 458 49 37
Fax 34 93 458 49 37
Email: jtizong@meditex.es

**ZAC DE FILC,** SARA Dr.
*Chair, Committee for Interregional Conferences*
*International Psychoanalytical Association*
Av., Las Heras 3855 - 6°piso
AR - 1425 Buenos Aires
Argentina
☎ 54 11 4802 2041
Fax 54 11 4802 2041
Email: sazacfilc@fibertel.com.ar

# Contents

## I. PSYCHOANALYSIS AND VIRTUAL REALITY



## II. PSYCHOSEXUALITY

## V. CONCLUSION

# Some Questions on Virtual Reality and Psychoanalysis

Jorge Canestri
*Italian Psychoanalytical Association*

The following notes and questions on the issue of virtual reality from a psychoanalytical point of view were written as an outline for an exchange of opinions at a round table. This is, therefore, not a paper about this theme, nor will these notes acquire any full meaning if they are separated from the other interventions. My intention during the round table was only that of setting some limits to the concept of 'virtual reality'. As it was an oral discussion, the bibliography refers only to the authors whose names are specifically mentioned.

There is a certain consensus concerning the fact that today there is an impact of 'artificialisation' on culture and social life, just like the impact of industrialisation in the $19^{th}$ century.

For many people the question is whether an artificial background that will become increasingly complex, can diminish our 'sense of reality'.

Are we conditioned by the idea that 'nature' is always good? Or at least that it is better than artificial products? And if so, why? Wooley proposed two hypotheses: a) because the 'natural order' operates within rhythms of evolution that are reassuring (natural selection works slowly), while technology alters these rhythms harshly; b) because, following the ethical principles of monotheistic religions, we presume that we cannot and must not receive «nothing in exchange for nothing». The principle of hubris is a correlate. But before discussing the excellence of nature as compared with invention, we must question the very concept of 'nature', as it proves to be as full of ideology as the concept of 'reality'.

There are two matters that need discussion before speaking of virtual reality and its impact on the mind and on culture; one is an ontological question: what is reality? The other is a gnoseological question, how can I know reality?

We have to acknowledge that even though reality has a consistency (here I accept a 'realistic' viewpoint in ontological terms, hence that reality is something that exists outside the subject and has a certain degree of independence from it), this consistency is far from being absolute. The concept of reality could be relativised from epistemological, sociological, linguistic, cultural and ideological points of view. Reality is not only something that 'consists', something that we could provisionally call 'real'; it is also a 'construction' that follows the needs and structure of the subject who knows. 'Virtual' reality is a particular manifestation, an expression of what I am calling 'reality', a 'special kind of reality'.

As a conclusion I could say that - even taking into account the usefulness of Occam's razor: «*Entia non sunt multiplicanda praeter necessitatem*» - it seems reasonable to accept that there are several kinds of 'reality' and that their nature merits careful reflection, above all if we seriously consider, to give one example, the challenge of quantum mechanics from an ontological and an epistemological viewpoint.

This is a very brief draft of the general problems raised by the concept of reality, but our main question on this occasion must be: what is the specificity of virtual reality? 'Virtual reality' depends on the existence of a special kind of machine that we have called a computer. All computers are a *simulation* of an ideal 'universal machine' that actualises the concepts mentioned by Alan Turing in 1937 in *On Computable Numbers*. All the things that a computer is able to do are *simulations.* Simulating is different from imitating. A simulation requires *an operative model*, an algorithm.

The two principles on which the construction of 'virtual reality' is based are: a) the use of pure mathematics to simulate real dynamics, and b) a device that allows men to interact with these simulations. What then is the nature of the objects that are the product of simulation? Are they fictitious? Imaginary? Real? They are 'mathematical objects'; they are the product of pure calculus, and have a particular kind of existence that we call 'virtual'. There is not a 'subject' of calculus (if not in the original construction of the program); calculus functions alone, it is automatic, and is the consequence of logical-mathematical syntax. The language of 'virtual reality' *is* the language of mathematics. Mathematical language is a symbolic one, but the product of simulation that interacts with men uses an iconic 'language'. This is one of the points we have to consider seriously - the continuous transformation of symbolic language into images.

This allows Baudrillard (1999, 2000) to postulate that the first stage of the sign and its use was that of being a reflex of reality; the second stage was that of the sign concealing reality, the third, that is the contemporary use of the sign in virtual reality, is that of pure simulation: *i.e.* the sign no longer means something real in the conventional sense - in a way, it is hyper-real.

We have here two issues that are significant for us as psychoanalysts for reflecting upon the effects of virtual reality on mental life. The first is the fact that the user is passive (while the creator of the program was active); he/she is the object in a certain sense of the automatic calculus. As the automatic calculus is itself without subject, because it is only the accomplishment of an algorithm, the subject is nowhere. The user is no longer the master but rather the slave of an automatic realisation. The second issue, as I have said above, concerns the transformation of symbolic language into iconic language (images). The continuous use of iconic language (that has an immediate reference to 'concrete' things; from this viewpoint it does not matter if things are 'real' or not) could seriously contribute towards the killing of thinking (in the French meaning of *pensée*) *and* imagination. Let us see why.

There are reasons linked to the machine (computer). A program, even a very sophisticated one, has no thinking. It may be 'intelligent', as in the case of 'expert systems', and solve difficult problems, but it does not think. Thinking is quite a different thing from intelligence, even though Turing disagrees (as do all the 'strong' IA). Here, I am considering thinking in the psychoanalytical terms of Bion, for example. As we know this implies the tolerance of frustration, of absence, and of 'negative realisations'. A necessary condition for the existence of thinking is the tolerance of the idea of 'no-thing', which means creating a place where a thought could be.

The impossibility of tolerating the idea of the 'no-thing' - that can be theorised as a deficit in the capacity for separatedness, for symbolisation, for tolerating and elaborating mourning, *etc.* - can result in the subject using the object (in our case the icon) to cancel the separation. This is one of the hypotheses of Ahumada (1999) about what Winnicott theorises as the transformation of the transitional object into the fetish object. Many authors (psychoanalysts as well as philosophers) insist on the de-mentalising, 'de-braining' effect of a certain type of use of the apparatuses of calculus. But that is where we must introduce some accurate distinctions between what is and what is not virtual reality, a topic about which, to tell the truth, considerable confusion exists both in psychoanalytic and in philosophic literature.

The continuous bombardment of images and icons that are of necessity stereotyped, and leave no space for thought, does not even leave space for imagination. In order to unfold, imagination needs *not* to be saturated with the repetitiveness of the realisation of the automatic calculus. And this is where the sense of impoverishment arises as the consequence of these experiences (from video games, as the most rudimentary expression, to virtual reality as the most complex realisation).

The most obvious consequence deriving from the compulsive use of virtual reality or from other forms of automatic calculus, even without the use of special interface devices, is the possibility of ignoring the existence of another 'reality', the reality of the Other, that can give rise to the total solipsism of the user. But this is a topic that is dealt with frequently.

To conclude I would like to mention two elements that could be counted among those that contribute to producing harmful effects on mental life. These points also display a coincidence between the psychoanalytic field and the field of philosophic thought. a) To change, *i.e.* to grow mentally is not the automatic consequence of receiving more information. Baudrillard believes that one can change (in the sense of introducing variants, what he calls 'morphisms') without becoming, without there being metamorphosis. The psychoanalytical reasons are to be found in Bion's above-mentioned theory of thinking. b) There is a problem relative to time: the automatic realisation of calculus allows for a certain atemporality, a certain repetitive and anhistoric contemporaneity.

I would like to emphasise that ascertaining the potential pathogenic effects of the computer's simulations in certain conditions of use does not mean denying the infinite possibilities offered by the realisation of automatic calculus. I think that a discussion on this theme should avoid either idealisation or demonisation. Both would reveal the ideological limitations and the ignorance that, unfortunately, have characterised most discussions on technique.

**References**

Ahumada, J.L., 1999, *Descubrimientos y refutaciones. La lógica de la indagación psicoanalítica*. Madrid, Ed. Biblioteca Nueva. Ch. 1.

Baudrillard, J., 1999, *L'Ëchange impossible*. Paris, Galilée.

Baudrillard, J., 2000, *Mots de passe*. Paris, Pauvert.

Turing, A., 1937, On Computable Numbers, with an Application to the Entscheidungsproblem, in: *Proceedings of the London Mathematical Society*, XLII, pp. 230-265.

Wooley, B., 1992, *Virtual Worlds*. Oxford, Blackwell Publishers.

# External Reality and Virtual Reality

Sara Zac de Filc
*Chair, Committee for Interregional Conferences, International Psychoanalytical Association*

## 1. SCIENCE AND TECHNOLOGY

The beginning of this new millennium is marked by great changes, especially in the fields of science and technology. This development has involved a vast expansion of information and communication technology, as well as molecular biology and biotechnology. We could say that the most representative milestone is the deciphering of the human genome. Our times, however, are also marked by the increase of anxiety and depression, by the lack of ability to delve into ourselves and devote to our minds the time and dedication they require.

Scientific and technological progress have basically brought about a transformation in the way we perceive time and space. We could say that speed has become a central component of our everyday world. The celerity of change forces us into a permanent awareness and exploration of new phenomena taking place in our societies, and to an ongoing in-depth study of our discipline. Only thus shall we be able to better understand the impact these transformations are having on human beings and, more specifically, on the human mind. In this sense, I believe that it is crucial to reflect upon the meaning of virtuality. In order to incorporate the changes it brings about not only in our perceptions but also in intersubjective relations, it is imperative to understand virtuality in all its senses. We must both assess its effects upon society and research its repercussion on the psyche. Thinking about virtuality takes us into a world that increasingly invades our surroundings. A new, apparent world arises, in which the borders between reality and fiction are blurred. An 'as if' emerges which produces spaces and times of simulation. These changes in our representations and perceptions of the surrounding world, raise serious problems in how we think about and face the new forms of development and how we might help to support the individual's personality, especially during periods which are themselves complex, such as early childhood and adolescence.

## 2. BUILDING THE EXTERNAL WORLD

In order to build the external world within him or herself, the individual incorporates his or her expectations based on past experiences, memories and unconscious fantasies of projected objects, in addition to perceptions of the objective world. Thus, personal relations are the key to identification and identity in the building of personality. The existence of virtual communication generates various spaces of relation which manifest themselves in the shape of an apparent game. In this game personality splitting, dissociations, role changes, parallel fantasmatic lives, and other phenomena may appear. These might bring about changes in one's way of thinking, in one's sexuality and identity. As Turkle puts it, it seems as if "besides making our work and communication easier, the computer offered us new models of the mind and a new medium where to project ideas and fantasies". In other words, it is as though the computer had become something more than a tool. It works as a mirror (though creating the illusion that we can go through it), in which our fantasies acquire a semblance of reality.

Cyberspace, the term used to describe virtual worlds, seems to allude to many real spaces. Born from science fiction, it is today, for many of us, a part of everyday routine. In cyberspace we may study, live, chat, read, and immerse ourselves. We should then ask ourselves how this new culture of parallel creation can affect our ideas about the mind, the body, and the relationship between the ego and the machine, the ego and others, the ego and the outer world.

In the context of these transformations, I would like to pose some questions I believe crucial for psychoanalysts. Does the use of simulators as the site for the projection of inner world fantasies produce new realities? To what extent does this production affect sensibility, perception, the here and now? What does it engender in the psyche? Does it lead to confusion?

## 3. IDENTITY AND THE «NEW» REALITIES

In the era of the Internet, virtual communities offer an entirely new context in which to think about human identity. They are spaces where we may learn directly about the meaning of a culture of simulation. An erosion of the limits between the real and the virtual, the animated and inanimate, the unitary and multiple ego, is taking place both in advanced scientific fields and in everyday life. We might have to ask ourselves what becomes of the ego when it divides its functions among the alterities which constitute it. Will the ego feel divided between separate worlds of virtuality and reality? Will the virtual world become a separate one in which people will get lost on other planes, or shall we learn the ways in which the real and the virtual may permeate each other while maintaining their potential for mutual enrichment and expansion? We must find ways to use virtuality that will not allow the veil of illusion that protects us from pain to lead us to unreality.

The imperative of self knowledge, always at the centre of philosophical research, also found expression in psychoanalytic culture. We work in order to get to know ourselves, so that we may improve not just our own lives but also those of our families and of the rest of our society. Psychoanalysis has evolved from its mechanicist, modernist roots, reaching new forms that are relevant for our times and cultures. Now is the time when we most need self-knowledge in order to render our lives significant, so that the screen will not replace the person within us.

We know, however, that the person and his or her ego are not passive entities determined by external forces. As I have stated before, the individual builds an outer world within from aspects of the objective world, from expectations based on past experiences, from memories and unconscious fantasies of objects, introjected and projected. The transformations of the ego's identity and its location in the world are aspects of a dialectic that determines that the changes occurring in a person are directly related to the bonds he/she creates. It is the expression of an inner world that is progressively built on the pillars that emerge in the early relationship of the child with its external and internal objects. This inner world constantly feeds off the external world and off relations established in the intrapersonal, the interpersonal and the transpersonal.

We look into this intimate realm in order to face the many-sided world in which the dialectic of cultural and technological changes marks us, affecting our subjectivity and leading to other dimensions of time and space, with the risk of disrupting the various spaces of perception. We must be creative and innovative, since we must rethink the way in which the inner and outer world relate, keeping in mind that these processes are closely bound to basic trust, which requires inner confidence. Such confidence rests on the possibility of metabolising death anxieties (Bion), or containing them (Winnicott) in such a way that new experiences might be assimilated.

Information technology and the changes in communication brought about by it raise problems of identity. The latter are connected to new forms of intersubjectivity which not only do not require the real other's presence, but also prevent us from identifying the other. That is the conundrum posited by virtuality. We have known since Freud that the erogenous body and the drive force are invariant. We also know that the thought generated in the non presence involves the possibility of fantasising about the absent object and projecting it again in one's mind. What happens to this process when the image is penetrated by another or others who invade it? What leads to the division of subjectivity into manifold egos and to playing with them? The other issue we must face as psychoanalysts is the possibility that virtuality will affect one's ability to come to terms with frustration. We might be led to feel that which has not been moulded in the real world has come to life on the screen. Only through further study within our discipline will we be able to face these dilemmas which increasingly demand that we go deeper into our science and that we learn in order to apprehend. An inner world that will enable us to identify with the internalised good objects will help us tolerate the vicissitudes of transition and overcome the anxiety generated by the temptation to split and to live in a virtual world only.

## 4. CONCLUSIONS

When we think of psychoanalysis and its spaces we know that through analysis a new, special virtuality is built between analyst and patient serving the rediscovery and liberation of the analysand's personality from the obstacles hindering his development. Moreover, we can also think of virtual space as one which opens up new options for inter- and trans-subjective bonds. How to make use of this virtuality? The answer to this question will be an important mission for psychoanalysis, and we will only be able to find it if we see virtuality not as a prison but as a space of transition in the search for freedom.

# Psychoanalysis and the New Technologies

Mauricio Gitnacht
*Swiss Psychoanalytical Society*

## 1. IS PSYCHOANALYSIS IN CRISIS?

We keep hearing that psychoanalysis is in a state of crisis. Well, I would like to begin by pointing out that psychoanalysis has always been controversial and always in a state of crisis. I do not want to discuss historical matters, but merely to refer briefly to the Victorian Era during which psychoanalysis was born and developed. From the end of the Second World War until roughly 1970, psychoanalysis had its glory days. But there was always, and I speak from personal experience, criticism of it, both explicit and implicit. It goes without saying that we always tried to minimise and rationalise these attacks, saying they were the offshoot of conflicts and the unconscious envy (and sometimes not as unconscious as all that) of the critic. Nevertheless, today, we are confronted by these attacks which have never ceased and which, on the contrary, have been renewed with a vigour which it is sometimes difficult to ward off. You know as well as I do that in Freud's time, he was faced with the hostility of his colleagues, as well as with rivalry and conflicts among his own disciples: Jung, Adler, Rank, Reich, *etc.* Each advanced his own theories, but I don't intend to document the history of psychoanalysis. I would like to address, at the dawn of the Third Millennium, the crisis psychoanalysis is faced with today and which concerns all of us. I shall try to do this, with a metapsychological outlook, using Freud's own ideas. In order to do this, I shall use as a starting point two articles by Freud, one written in 1927: *The Future of an Illusion* and the other in 1930: *Civilization and its Discontents*. In these articles, Freud expresses himself more in relation to the multiple interests of psychoanalysis, such as, for example, the natural sciences, philosophy and culture in general. Effectively, he had already written about these topics in his article entitled *Totem and Taboo* in 1912.

He also addressed the similarities and differences between illusions and delirium. But the concept of the reality principle remains the most important element to differentiate between them, despite the difficulties implicit in their definition. For him, the only path capable of leading us into reality, external to ourselves, was scientific research.

In his article *The Future of an Illusion*, Freud addressed problems linked to culture, to civilisation and their impact on the psyche. He asked questions about their influence on implied narcissistic satisfaction which forces the renunciation of instinctive imperatives. In other words, imposing the reality principle onto the pleasure principle with all the related consequences. Man has an illusion: to master the forces of nature, Freud told us, but we are confronted by reality and our own impotence. And while we may sometimes believe in this illusion, there is at least one aspect which escapes man, this is the enigma of our mortality which forces us to face our inherent weakness, our experience of profound impotence when confronted by this reality and its corollary, a feeling of «helplessness» (*Hilflösigkeit*) which we first experienced at birth - our first contact with reality.

Man, said Freud, then calls upon the gods who, and I quote: «retain their threefold task: they must exorcise the terrors of nature, they must reconcile men to the cruelty of Fate, particularly as it is shown in death, and they must compensate them for the sufferings and privations which a civilised life in common has imposed on them». Freud concluded that MOIRA (fate) is imposed even on the gods, as they themselves have their own destiny. But that is insufficient for men to rid themselves of their feelings of «helplessness» (*Hilflösigkeit*).

From that point on, we discovered a Freud who was almost, I would say, a mystic, who calls upon a unique superior force, infinite and all-powerful. But Freud extricated himself from a tight metaphysical spot, by adding that this implied a return to the childhood necessity of seeing in the father's face the unique and all-powerful being who will defend his child against feelings of «helplessness». Freud will give religions the same values that they bestow on civilisation, that of mastering the forces of nature. In this context, he turned dialectical and polemical. For him, an illusion is the result of a childish desire.

«It is once again merely an illusion to expect anything from intuition and introspection» wrote Freud. He admitted to being an atheist. For him, all religious doctrine had to be illusion. This hasn't prevented some of our colleagues, even today, from considering psychoanalysis as a religion. Freud said: it is an illusion. But the fundamental concepts of psychoanalysis: the existence of the unconscious, the reality of infantile sexuality and transference, are not illusions. They have been subjected to the test of reality. Freud continues to grow in depth where the links to, and contradictions in civilisations, cultures, sciences and religions are concerned. He was opposed to the premise that the decline of religion was the product of scientific advances and feared that the same arguments would be used to discredit psychoanalysis. Don't we find ourselves, 70 years later, at the same point? Freud indulged in dialectics himself to conclude that the goal of psychoanalysis is to master the world of instinct. He insisted strongly on the destructive instincts of man and took as an example the desire to kill, which he attributed in a historical perspective to parricide which could be controlled by a fear of an all-powerful God and not by reason. For Freud, and I quote: «Religion would thus be the universal obsessional neurosis of humanity; like the obsessional neurosis of children, it arose out of the Oedipus complex, out of the relation to the father».

Psychoanalysis frightens in the same way freedom does. Dictatorships and dictators fear both. To put us into contact with our unconscious, to remove repression and confront us with our Oedipal complex implies facing up to our world of instinct. This is frightening; we are frightened of losing control over our instincts and falling into chaos. From there, it is easy to deduce the confusion certain people feel between freedom and chaos (madness).

## 2. PSYCHOANALYSIS AND THE NEW PSYCHOTHERAPIES

Freud stated that psychoanalysis was a science and therefore a source of knowledge. But today, this is not taken for granted. Psychoanalysis as a science is under debate. As I already mentioned, certain people consider it to be a religion. From this arose a rush to carry out research on psychoanalysis while forgetting, insofar as Freud was concerned, that psychoanalysis was research in and of itself. The neurosciences, technological exploits, biology, cybernetics, genetics and so on, gained the upper hand vis-à-vis psychoanalysis as a science.

Other psychotherapeutic techniques appeared and competed with psychoanalysis; you are familiar with them. There were systemic therapies, cognitive, behavioural and I have just learned of a new therapeutic technique which we have imported; dialectic cognitive therapy which is intended to specifically treat borderline patients. Well, why not? ... but psychoanalysis will remain, in my view, a science which has proved its worth and will continue, in the spirit of scientific research and in collaboration with other sciences, to grow richer and more fully developed. It is true that certain people endowed psychoanalysis with a miracle-worker dimension. This was only, of course, an illusion. We know full well the therapeutic limits to psychoanalysis, but this doesn't prevent us from recognising the results of research carried out in this framework. Metapsychology as a methodology for the understanding of the functioning of the psyche has been and is still debated. In these instances, nothing nor anyone, till now, has been able to replace Freudian metapsychology.

## 3. PSYCHOANALYSIS AND TECHNOLOGICAL ADVANCES

At the dawn of the Third Millennium, we find ourselves confronted by important changes in the fields of science, and technology which influence the environment, including humankind. People must, therefore, adapt themselves psychologically, economically and socially. These efforts at adaptation provoke anxiety, reactionary depressions and sometimes confused states. The tendency would be to find rapid relief: «we never have the time». Benzodiazepines, anti-depressants and neuroleptics have made a lightening eruption into our daily lives. I am not opposed to them, but they will never replace the work of introspection, nor psychoanalytical investigation which might lead to a better knowledge of one's self and a refurbishment of our interior lives. The magic pill remains to be discovered, just as does the «happiness pill» to prevent the suffering with which we are often confronted on the difficult road of psychoanalysis. A road which is built out of replacing instantaneous gratification (which corresponds to functioning on the model of the pleasure principle) by the reality principle. Another example of this would be the myriad semi-religious cults which propose accession to an «easy and uncomplicated paradise». Reality is, of course, very different.

Despite technological progress, humanity still yearns for happiness. I will quote here what Freud said in 1930 in *Civilization and its Discontents*: «During the last few generations mankind has made an extraordinary advance in the natural sciences and in their technical application and has established his control over nature in a way never before imagined. The single steps of this advance are common knowledge and it is unnecessary to enumerate them. Men are proud of those achievements, and have a right to be. But they seem to have observed that this newly-won power over space and time, this subjugation of the forces of nature, which is the fulfilment of a longing that goes back thousands of years, has not increased the amount of pleasurable satisfaction which they may expect from life and has not made them feel happier.»

## 4. THE DEMANDS OF THE 21ST CENTURY PATIENT

Instantaneous gratification (infantile) is the demand. The mechanisms of repression are missing. Aggressiveness and destructiveness are manifested with a permissiveness that could never have been imagined before, spreading at the speed of the new means of communication, and even globalisation. Freud proposed the sublimation of instincts to put a break on our instinctive drives and through this, the possibility of satisfaction thanks to mental and intellectual work. I quote him: «A satisfaction of this kind, such as an artist's joy in creating, in giving his fantasies body, or a scientist's in solving problems or discovering truths, has a special quality which we shall certainly one day be able to characterise in metapsychological terms.» Freud is far from proposing sublimation as an ideal solution, but he gives it pride of place among others.

We cannot stop scientific technological progress, nor can we, in our role as psychoanalysts, prevent its repercussions on our understanding of the human being's evolution and on the degree to which we can try to find a metapsychological explanation, as Freud suggested himself.

My observations have given me the impression that new discoveries and new techniques push individuals towards a disengagement with instinct to the detriment of inhibition, towards narcissistic satisfaction to the detriment of the relation with the object and toward destructiveness to the detriment of the libido: the interactive to the detriment of the inter-subjective.

## 5. A CLINICAL EXAMPLE

At this stage, I would like to mention the case of the young woman who was referred to me with a diagnosis of serious depression which did not respond to anti-depressants. The patient in question was an agreeable, well-groomed young woman of 28 but who, the minute she sat down and without my asking her a single question, began crying and couldn't stop. After several minutes, she calmed down a little. She told me then that she was a secretary and that for the past several months, almost a year, she had been surfing the Internet for several hours each day. Between sobs, she told me that she had met - via the Internet - many people. She had made friends (?) but she couldn't stop surfing. She is married, childless and told me her marriage was suffering from her addiction. Her husband was very understanding. She had not been able to sleep for several months. Then she started to cry again and added: «I can't take it anymore».

After this first discussion, I asked myself questions about this patient and I felt very divided as to a diagnosis. All I saw was a woman who was confused and invaded by anxiety, with an adolescent personality... borderline?

During the three subsequent discussions, she explained to me how, behind the anonymity of a computer screen, she let herself (regress) expressing her most archaic (erotic) fantasies to her invisible partners. Fantasies of flagellation, bondage... in other words, an excess of sado-masochistic fantasies had irrupted in her life and invaded a great part of her psyche, which she had great difficulty in controlling. But the possibility of expressing herself in front of me seemed to calm her. She wept less and became more capable of communicating without feeling threatened. Her ego, on the brink of breakdown because of a superego which had become sadistic, gave me the impression of wanting to gain the upper hand.

She told me that when she was little, she was subjected to fondling by her father, but when she complained about this to her mother, the mother minimised things or changed the subject. She spoke to me about her husband who did not understand her, was completely passive and incapable of satisfying her (erotic) fantasies. She seemed more at ease.

At the beginning of our fourth session, sobbing, she told me she had something else to tell me, while she fidgeted in her armchair. She told me that several months before, following a contact made on the Internet, she was asked by one of her partners to meet in a pre-determined location, which she accepted. Once there, she gave in to all his demands. She was beaten, tied up, handcuffed, *etc.* and at a certain moment, she became frightened and managed to escape, covered in bruises, and wounded.

During her story, with tears in her eyes, she kept her eyes on me to gauge my reactions. I admit I was very touched by her story. But as soon as her story was over, she began to cry again saying: «but you know, I liked it. I'm afraid I'm going to do it again.» I could not prevent myself from asking her the question: are you still in contact with these men? A resounding «yes and that frightens me». After this confession, she became confused and I had great difficulty in re-establishing contact.

As I thought this over, I asked myself some questions:

1. what sort of relationship did this woman establish with the very first objects to which she related and how did she organise them in her psyche?

2. what were the consequences for the organisation of her early ego and superego, as well as in their reciprocal relationships?

3. what role did memories of the father's incestuous fondling (real or fantasised) play in the current symptomatology of the patient?

4. what is the importance of the computer/Internet, as an intermediate object, in setting off this pathology?

5. how was this organised from a metapsychological point of view?

Freud said: «Experience shows, however, that the severity of the superego which a child develops in no way corresponds to the severity of treatment which he has himself met with (as has been rightly emphasised by M. Klein and other English writers)».

My patient felt torn between the demands of the world of instinct (her id), her ego and her superego. We can think that this structure springs from a permissive environment which lacks containment. All this results in the emergence of a «conscience» like the one my patient revealed. The innate factor has also played an important role. The influence of these new technologies: do they have a real impact in the sense that they promote the appearance of new psychic structures? Yes and no. In my opinion, they only work as intermediary objects of another type. They offer us the possibility of accessing the realisation of our most archaic fantasies by disorganising the process of inhibition. This disorganisation is going to allow the reappearance of perverse, polymorphic infantile aspects of the past.

The perverted affect present in the subject's relationships with the new objects produced by these new technological discoveries, is going to provoke internal conflicts. The result could be mental dysfunction, as in the case of my patient, in which the computer (and its functions) played the role of a parasite which would risk confusing the individual who lacks appropriate defences. The «conscience» and the reality principle are in danger. I would use the same terms to express myself in relation to the virtual world that is revealed to us by these new technologies.

Will new generations be better prepared to face these challenges? And how will we, as psychoanalysts, confront these new technological developments from the topographic, economic and dynamic points of view? Or can a new metapsychology be imagined? My opinion is that as the individual remains the same, we should adapt or integrate Freudian metapsychology, which is always valid, to parry this challenge.

As long as the patient had not acted upon her fantasies, she could manage to confront her feelings of guilt. But once she had acted upon them, guilt overcame her and turned into remorse, as Freud would say. She was no longer capable of defending herself and this guilt no longer had any value from an economic standpoint.

From a dynamic point of view, we could say that the patient used the computer as an intermediary to enact punishment on herself for her unconscious guilt subsequent to incestuous relations with her father.

## 6. CONCLUSIONS

It seems to me that the new civilisation with which we are confronted, is showing itself to be more permissive, but just as restrictive. Will illusions become reality? I am personally convinced that the internal world of future generations will be confronted by the same problems and conflicts as we are today. So much so, that we should adapt ourselves to the new models of identification and relations with the object, produced as a result of scientific progress such as genetic manipulation, cloning and various forms of fertilisation which raise issues about the concept of identity: ours as well as those of our patients.

Freud described the ego as being a headlong rush towards identification. This is also valid for the superego. What identifications will men use as a basis for their future? How will they evolve? And the id? I think that it will continue to be the container of the world of instinct.

**References**

Freud, S., 1912, *Totem and Taboo*, standard edition
Freud, S., 1927, *The Future of an Illusion*, standard edition
Freud, S., 1930, *Civilization and its Discontents*, standard edition

# A Psychoanalyst: Between an Excess of the Virtual and an Excess of Realism

Jean-Michel Quinodoz
*Training Analyst, Swiss Psychoanalytic Society*

## 1. «WHY CAN'T I GRAB IT?»

I would like to talk about virtual reality by telling you a true story. One day, a little boy I shall call Jacques came to see us and asked me: «May I take the pretty little pink pig I can see on the bookshelf? I'd like to play with it». I replied: «Yes, you may try». Jacques approached it with his hand, closing his fingers around the object and shouted with surprise: «But there's no little pig! I can't touch it!» In fact, his fingers were clutching air. Jacques' face became sad, his voice expressed his disappointment and worry: «But I can see it! Why can't I grab it?» Jacques remained motionless, showing some anxiety.

To alleviate his frustration, I opened the box above which the virtual little pig could be seen and I took out the real one, the one placed on the focus of a concave mirror. I put it in Jacques' hand and he squeezed it tightly, as if he did not want it to escape. He said to me, with a huge smile of relief: «It's really real this little pig which wasn't real!» After a short silence, Jacques was once again seized by the wish to play and asked: «But then, where's the other one, the one I couldn't grab?»

## 2. FROM «VIRTUAL OR REAL» TO «VIRTUAL AND REAL»

What can we learn from this story? Firstly, I would say that in order to draw someone's attention to a virtual object, you need to choose an object which will particularly awaken the interest of that person. This happened with Jacques who was attracted to the little pig he wanted to play with, and for this reason he felt frustrated and disappointed. Then Jacques was troubled because he felt trapped in an alternative in which each aspect was as troubling as the other: either he is disappointed at not being able to touch a little pig which has no reality and escapes; or he squeezes a real little pig in his hand which he does not want to escape. In either case, Jacques feels worried and troubled, to the point where playing with the little pig suddenly loses all its charm ...

However, a moment later, Jacques pulled himself together when he realised that the little pig that he was holding in his hand might exist elsewhere, and started to search for it, saying: «But where's the other one ...?» The charm worked again because Jacques was then able to emerge from the two alternatives of either totally virtual, or totally real. In his mind he was able to create a link between the real object *and* the virtual object, a link which distinguishes and connects both, according to a process analogous to the creation of symbols which gives access to symbolic representation. In fact I think it is the same for the virtual as for the symbolic, the latter being based on a tripartite relation: the symbol, the symbolised object, and the person for whom the symbol becomes the symbol of the object (H. Segal, 1991). Any disturbances arising in this tripartite relation, carry with them disturbances in the function of symbolism, as in that of virtual reality.

## 3. TRANSFERENCE: VIRTUAL REALITY AND REAL REALITY

We can now ask ourselves: isn't it the same with the transference relationship between patient and psychoanalyst? In order for the «charm» of the transference to work, it is crucial that this relationship takes place in an area which is neither totally virtual nor totally real, but both virtual *and* real. This is an unstable equilibrium, which modifies itself from one moment to the next, necessitating a constant balancing act in order to integrate the two extremes (J.M. Quinodoz, 1991). If there is a tendency towards too much virtual reality or, conversely, towards too much reality, there is a risk of too much distancing from the specific field of psychic reality, and of endangering the transference relationship between patient and psychoanalyst.

Let's take the example of feelings the patient has in relation to the psychoanalyst. It may happen that a patient takes the psychoanalyst as a purely virtual person and addresses him as if he doesn't exist: «Here, you are a psychoanalyst. For me you are not a real person, therefore I can tell you anything, even the nastiest things, and this will not affect you!» or: «At any rate, I am not angry with you as a person. You are not my mother!» Here the patient suffers from being with a purely virtual psychoanalyst who has no feelings. On the contrary, it may happen that a patient becomes persuaded that he/she is in love with or detests the real person of the psychoanalyst. At that moment he/she feels endangered, fearing that the psychoanalyst's feelings might reciprocate his or her own.

Where is the psychoanalyst to be situated as an object of transference, and where is the person of the psychoanalyst with his/her own, true sensitivity? Herein lies the art of the psychoanalyst: it consists of maintaining a delicate balance between the feelings produced by the virtual phenomenon of transference and the feelings towards the real person.

## 4. A DANGER WHICH COMES FROM PSYCHOANALYSTS THEMSELVES?

This delicate balance has to be maintained by the psychoanalyst on two levels. The psychoanalyst aims to maintain it on the *individual* level of the transferential relationship between patient and psychoanalyst. He or she also aims to maintain it on a *collective* level in such a way that the practice of psychoanalysis remains viable in the framework of contemporary society. On the collective level as well as on the individual level, this constitutes a delicate balance that is often threatened not only from forces exterior to psychoanalysis but also sometimes from within. That is to say by psychoanalysts themselves who risk putting the survival of a viable psychoanalysis in danger, either by according too great an importance to what is virtual, or, on the contrary, to what is real. I would like to add a few more words about this before concluding.

## 5. FROM RUNNING THE RISK OF AN EXCESS OF VIRTUAL REALITY…

I shall start with the risk of an excess of virtual reality. For example, if you push the notion of intersubjectivity too far, and you place the analytical exchange in an area which belongs neither to the patient nor to the analyst, don't you run the risk of transforming the psychoanalytical process into a purely virtual and disembodied phenomenon? And this may especially happen, to my mind, if you start from this conceptualisation of the transference to conclude that the psychoanalytical process remains the same whatever the conditions of its setting. I see another excess of virtual reality in the idea that the psychoanalytical cure would only be suitable for neurotic patients. Why? Because I think that if psychoanalysis were to be considered as suitable only for those persons who attain a good level of mental functioning, would be to ignore the possibilities offered by current technical psychoanalysis to enable a large category of patients - who are dominated by concrete thought - to slowly but surely gain access to symbolic functions thanks to a psychoanalytical treatment.

## 6. ...TO RUNNING THE RISK OF AN EXCESS OF REALISM

And what about the risk of an excess of realism on the part of the psychoanalyst? In this respect, I see the threat to psychoanalysis of soon – if not already - being replaced by new pharmaceutical medications as well as by new discoveries from the field of the neurosciences. I also see the risk of an excess of realism when one tries to capture transferential phenomena so as to objectify and prove that psychoanalysis has a true scientific basis. For example, the tape recording of a session remains for me as illusory as trying to grasp a virtual image with the hand in order to ascertain that it exists.

I also see the psychoanalyst running the risk of an excess of realism in the idea that shorter therapies with one or two sessions a week, face to face, would result in the development of a transference process identical to that of psychoanalysis, which necessitates four to five sessions a week, with the patient lying on a couch.

## 7. CONCLUSION

I have been working as a psychoanalyst for more than thirty years, and I can tell you that, in contact with my analysands, I rediscover everyday the extent to which psychoanalysis has kept its full strength and vigour, even one hundred years after having been created. Moreover, daily experience has shown me that far more patients could in fact benefit from a psychoanalytical treatment as long as the analysts themselves maintain sufficient confidence in its value to keep it on offer - today as in the past.

Nowadays many of my contemporaries - among them many psychoanalysts - consider me as a Utopian who ignores today's realities, especially the realities of the third millennium. I agree that I may appear Utopian, but personally feel I am as much a realist as a Utopian: I feel I am sufficiently realistic to account for the conditions that need to be met for a true psychoanalytic process to be properly realised, at the same time I feel I am sufficiently Utopian to believe in a reality which cannot be held in your hand...

**References**

Quinodoz, J.M., 1991, *The Taming of Solitude. Separation Anxiety in Psychoanalysis*. Transl. Ph. Slotkin. London and New York: Routledge, 1993
Segal, H., 1991, *Dream, Phantasy and Art*. London and New York: Routledge

# Castration, an Illusory Virtual Reality

Olivier Flournoy
*Swiss Psychoanalytical Society*

## 1. THE CHALLENGES OF THE INTERNET

The Internet has revolutionised everything, up to and including the idea of «real life» or, for us, sexual identity.

In a millennium past (which was - in reality - only a year ago), a chess player pitted his wits against the artificial intelligence of an IBM, Big Blue. A clash of «titans». Would the computer with its lightning speed and the billions of connections and program instructions with which it was endowed by hundreds of talented information technologists, rob the human brain (and its billions of synapses) of its throne, finally asserting the supremacy of machine over man and cognitivists over psychoanalysts?

But this did not take into consideration the Internet. Because of the Web, that same human chess player, using his or her screen as a chessboard, can take part in games in cyberspace, directly defying the skill of IBM's greatest minds, while grafting onto their expertise the individual's own intelligence, own capacity for self-analysis, own feelings, passions, enthusiasms or fears, as well as his or her whims: in short all those things that a computer cannot do.

By repudiating this duel of gladiators, it is possible to embrace a culture of communication and negotiation where men and women can finally meet on an equal footing. And we can no longer reply to the dilemma arising from the question «who am I?» by an unequivocal response: male, female...or machine.

Surfing the Internet transforms concepts of reality and of gender. If I decide, while sitting in front of my screen and writing to my correspondents all over the world, to modify my appearance, change my weight, my height, my age, the colour of my eyes, and even my gender, there's nothing to stop me. For example, I can present myself as a young man or young woman who loves this or that and who, naturally, weaves a web around the world, constituting a virtual community but who also creates a network of very real, interested parties to befriend, with whom I will enter into discussions, exchanges, indulge in sexual adventures, *etc.*, even if I refuse to meet them in person. And the psychoanalyst knows full well to what extent psychosexuality lends itself to this type of relationship. The boundaries between fantasy and reality dissolve; the physical body is no longer the guarantor of «reality». And, by putting aside the physical side of these relationships - no risk of intercourse, pregnancy, rape, venereal diseases, AIDS, aggression...- the affects, the emotions become uninhibited, are released as if under a magnifying glass. Here again, the similarities between cybernetic and psychoanalytic dialogue are manifest. Just as the chat room visitors can become suddenly and violently jealous of an anonymous cyberfriend, analysands and analysts know full well that the feelings they may experience towards each other often go beyond what they feel in real life.

The fact that simulation precedes and foreshadows reality is certainly nothing new, but today interface relationships between surfers come accompanied by a coefficient of objective/subjective reality such as is conferred onto intertransferential relationships as they are lived in analysis. What I mean is this: in chat rooms the simulated relationship (a cyber-correspondent introduces him- or herself as he or she pleases and not as he or she is) leads to real affects. And in the case of analysis, a fantasmatic relationship, mother/son for instance, between the two participants leads to real feelings. Thus an unprecedented equation is added on, tending to erase the boundaries between fantasy and reality and between the sexes. Like the analyst who may, in the transference, become mother, father, *etc.*, whatever his or her real gender and identity, the cybergeek may change his or hers at whim.

These changes in identity have led distinguished female writers (Odzer, 1997; Palac, 1998; Turkle, 1997) who have experimented with cybersex to draw some remarkable conclusions: real life is composed of males and females and - this is the interesting point - no value judgment can be made about the superiority of one over the other. These women are women and their female characteristics, they say, can in no way be devalourised or overvalourised vis-à-vis the males. For instance, the so-called sexual passivity of women is in no way synonymous with inferiority. And to be more explicit, a clitoris is neither better nor worse than a penis. Here a value judgment has no meaning; it is absurd. For us psychoanalysts, this means that the female's anatomical gender is not characterised by the lack of a penis, nor the male's by the lack of a uterus. We are faced here with an egalitarian value judgment between males and females – no machismo, no masochism - which, to me, seems unusual and promising.

Adding this new card to the deck, I propose examining two concepts, two psychoanalytical models which no longer fit into the scheme of things, as I was taught them: castration and the mother-child couple. Both effectively give rise to the question of where to draw the line between reality and fantasy.

According to traditional psychoanalysis and the castration complex theory, reality implies a virtual phallicised/castrated couple with implications for the body itself. The boy would be morphologically phallicised and threatened with castration, the girl would be anatomically castrated. In my opinion, such a distinction is no longer valid. The inequality and the disharmony to which this image bears witness is based on a fallacious representation of anatomy as such, a fantasy-representation taken literally (what is real is not a fantasised lack of a penis, but female sex characteristics: clitoris, vagina, *etc.*). Girls and boys are different but complementary, to each his or her own gender from birth, and the supremacy of the male based on the so-called castration or real absence of a penis in the little girl is a fantasy with no anatomical basis.

Thus, equality from the start between women and men could become one of the greatest acquisitions of the dawning century and psychoanalysis could have the merit of being a pioneer in this regard.

As far as the psychoanalytic mother/child couple is concerned - the focus of so much work and so many expectations, the same story applies. As virtual as it might be, it is also based on a fictitious reality: it is obvious that if the mother had simply been a child, she could belong to either gender or to neither, just like the child who is of no particular gender. This gives her a staggering responsibility and reduces the importance of the father to hardly anything. The mother must find her place as the woman who can only give birth to boys or girls, as a mother who can only become one if copulation has taken place with the future father and if she has herself been a girl and not a boy.

The virtual «mother/child entity»only exists if she also represents this reality made up of men and woman and of newborns, male or female.

Once castration is freed from morphology's mastery which prevented it from being a psychoanalytical illusory virtual reality, *i.e.* a fantasy, and once the «mother/child» entity is freed from the domination of its fictitious but so-called real nature which also prevented it from becoming a psychoanalytical illusory virtual reality, *i.e.* a fantasy, any analyst, man or woman, can live out with his or her subject - male or female- a fantasised, *i.e.* virtual, phallic/castrated or mother/child entity in the transference relationship, both being variations of the Oedipus complex.

The equality of the sexes is ensured by innate differences.

## 2. CASTRATION AND THE MOTHER/CHILD ENTITY

There is a link between the Freudian concept of castration and the post-Freudian concept of the «mother-child» entity. Both are illusory virtual realities, fantasies. The analyst and his analysand are realities. They see each other, talk and listen to each other, shake hands. Virtuality concerns the transference, an illusory virtuality. The transference's imaginings will never become realities. Virtual reality concerns the analytic couple whose dialogue stems from transference and countertransference, a virtuality included in a relative reality, without physical contact, but a virtuality which is real indeed as shown by affects, more than often violent, overwhelming, inescapable, which are felt on both sides, and through discourse and its frequent misunderstandings.

Castration is a virtual reality although illusory. It frightens, it paralyses, but as far as I know, it has never been acted out by an Oedipal father on his son's penis, and never has a girl been castrated, deprived of a penis. Long before her birth, she has a clitoris and female sex organs. As a matter of fact, children, whatever their sex, can behave in a phallic or castrated mode, feel sexually aroused or not, long before the parental threat materialises. The «bedrock» is indeed sex and gender for both. There should be no value judgment about some male attributes which the female lacks.

The mother-child couple is also an illusory virtual reality. Even before birth each child is girl or boy, and only girls will become mothers. After conception, this real and mythical instant uniting two and three people where the gender of the being conceived is still unknown, the foetus gets its own sexual identify, independent of the parent who does not share it. A thought-provoking hypothesis developed recently suggests the possible suicide (Apoptosis) of those cells bearing the characteristics of the gender lost at conception (Ameisen, 1999).

Birth corroborates the fact that the mother does not give birth to a child: when the child appears, the mother does not ask: «is it a child?» a terrifying question indeed, but «is it a baby boy, a baby girl?» An important question, since the mother, having been a baby girl, will relate differently to a girl than to a boy who will never become a mother. Thus, the traditional mother-child concept denies the child the gender it has missed out on, and denies that the mother lacks the father's gender. And it denies the mother her own gender inasmuch as she would never have been a baby girl herself, but simply a child. Witnesses at birth confirm: the birth of a 'child' is an illusion, a negation of its gender: as the head appears they don't say that it is a child, not a monster, they hold their breath until they see the gender and acknowledge the birth of a girl or a boy. Here, the English expressions 'baby boy' or 'baby girl' are perfectly relevant.

To deny the infant its gender absolves it and places the burden of sin on the mother who monopolises it while, simultaneously, it robs her of her sexuality. She becomes a non-sexual monster, totally responsible for her child's future. An absence of the mother, for just a bit too long, may lead her child to fall into an unthinkable abyss of helplessness and terror leading eventually to psychosis. If this occurs because of the absence of a father or a nurse, they will not be held responsible because they are mere substitutes. We should renounce such a value judgment and substitute for mother-child entity that of parent-child, or that of mother/father-baby boy or baby girl, which are the three sides of the Oedipal triangle.

## 3. CASTRATION, GIRLS AND BOYS

Freud has always maintained that the acknowledgment of castration or the dread of castration takes place in a deferred way. In 1909, for instance, little Hans perceives and notices that some living beings have no penis, and remains interested in sexual matters without inhibition and without even taking castration's threats seriously until a particular day when the parent's or the mother's threat scares him. One does not know why the threat was taken seriously on that particular day and why only then castration was linked to the representation of the female genitals, considered as nothing more than a missing penis. Towards the end of his life, in 1938, Freud introduced the concept of the splitting of the ego and suggested that this happens when the castration threat has been uttered in an extremely violent way by a woman speaking in the name of the father. The child in question is a boy who misses a little girl with whom he had shared exciting sexual games, and who, deprived of his little friend's presence, sinks into a frenzy of masturbation.

The adult threat, a hazardous cultural occurrence, even if it is the mother screaming warnings in the name of the father, is manifestly insufficient to trigger the castration complex. The seeds must have been planted in ground that was furrowed by desire and curiosity for an object endowed with genitals different from his, a necessary precondition to set the stage for the anxiety which leads to repression. Or else in ground made barren by frustration due to the lack of this sexually arousing object which leads to the splitting of the ego. The little boy in 1938 must have kept the memory of a little girl endowed with true feminine genitals which his mother's threat caused him to transform into a false representation: 'this girl must have been a castrated boy', a way of making the threat real while, by the same token, justifying it. In altering his representation, the boy negates the adult's lie and transforms it into a truth. What appears significant here is the weight of reality given by Freud to castration: the boy first perceives the female genitals, is interested and aroused by them, but without consequences. He then does not repress this reality but the representation of a castrated male sex organ - neurosis - or the denial of this representation - splitting.

Contrary to Freud's opinion, nothing whatsoever allows us to think that the boy, when he played with or looked at the little girl's genitals saw anything else than a girl with female sex organs. The concept of castration - a fact for the girl and a threat or even a negative hallucination for the boy - is thus grounded in a child's false representation conveyed by an adult's lie, which is a false cultural and intentional representation. And from then on, from this little boy's representation, with the participation of the adults, all psychoanalytical children are split into two categories: those who dread castration, the future men, and those who are castrated of their penis, the future women. Furthermore castration as a 'so-called' fact is upheld by the 1938 paper in which the faulty perception itself is denied in order to keep the idea of a non-castrated object: thus a non-castrated girl is a boy's fantasy built on a false representation, that is on a boy without a penis. Therefore a non-castrated girl does not exist; she is a boy.

I believe this attitude to be totally outdated. Culturally, castration (eunuch, castrato) differs from the complex. As for the girl, she could well be threatened just like the boy: 'stop it or you will never grow breasts', a displacement upwards (never have a vagina) which points to the mother/child entity, and a threat which might deprive her of her charms or attraction, narcissistic or object related. The threat of castration, by whoever, father or mother or their representatives, once uttered and registered leads to the same aberrations: one could be castrated or one is castrated whatever one's gender. Castration is an illusory virtual reality, a fantasy and not a normal constituent of the psyche. This constituent which structures or builds it is the Oedipal complex. If real, castration would mean a mutilation of the genitals. If virtually real, the threat of the adults could become reality. Now, this never occurs in psychoanalysis: it is illusory. As a matter of fact, it never happens at all: if a father cuts off the penis of his son, that makes him neither a girl nor a castrato, just a cripple.

Castration implies a false appreciation of the genders, which leads to a disparaging judgment towards females. Castration is a psychic illusion which, according to Freudian theory, unfortunately rests on an absence of female penises, on a nothingness, eventually on a disparagement of female sexuality. In comparison, if the dream is a psychic illusion, it implies sleep, otherwise it wouldn't be a dream. And it becomes a virtual reality once included in the analytic dialogue, whatever the gender of the sleeper. The dream in psychoanalysis, whether uttered or not, leads to the reality of the unconscious and of the undesirable desire.

It would be interesting to question ourselves about the first representation of the child's perception leading to the castration complex, the perception of the genitals which the child does not have. Here Freud is ambiguous: the child does not react, does not care, but nevertheless it arouses him. What he sees becomes a mnemonic trace. As far as the boy is concerned, he literally does not see anything, he sees nothing. And this is not considered as an error but as reality: there is nothing to look at. And many analysts agree. They consider that on the girl's side there is nothing to see because what there is to see is hidden, or even worse because a split means nothing, a hole is nothing...a hole without rims? In my opinion we are here confronted with an adult interpretation of the primal perception of the female genitals by a boy. And this is Freud's interpretation, the interpretation of a repressing adult. Such interpretation absolves the child. But which child? Little Hans, the boy. And of course it absolves the adult as well.

The supposedly unconcerned child can be retraced when a boy or a girl, looking at genitals speaks of «wee-wees» as if eager to absolve him- or herself of being sexually aroused in order to please the adult. Plainly speaking, the boy has a tap, a pipe, the girl has none, but both urinate nevertheless. And yet the libido is still at work: both Freud's boys (Hans and the one mentioned in 1938) have perceived the strangeness of sex, an endless source of curiosity and excitement leading to masturbation.

For girls and boys, obviously, sexual investigation arises from the discovery of the genitals, authentic objects of desire, before any castration fantasy. Whereas, for instance, in relation to breasts, all children are identical, jealous of each other; they are all clones whatever their gender.

Viewing with 'libidinal eyes' the female or the male genitals - nothing like a penis, missing or not - should certainly be the precondition of the anxiety which follows the threat. Can one «see» without libidinal cathexis? One should say yes, of course. But if so the psychoanalyst has to choose: either the boy views the female sex organ with an aroused libidinally cathected and pleasurable look and what he has seen becomes unpleasurably cathected in a deferred way at the time of the threat, or he sees nothing according to the parent's wish and the threat becomes unintelligible. The perception of the genitals which one does not possess constitutes therefore the first step leading to the castration fantasy.

With Freudian theory, we are faced with an adult's denial: when the adult says that the first perception of the girl's genitals does not affect the boy, he negates the fact that the boy has seen a non-ego since he keeps a mnemonic trace or a vivid memory of the event. He absolves the child: 'is it a baby boy or a baby girl? No, it is a suckling infant', is what adults say, implying that all children must be similar, identical, clones, half of whom have been mutilated and denominated as girls. This Freudian non-perception or non-reaction of a child confronted with a child whose genitals are not the same, is thus a memory trace belonging to the adult who transforms for his or her convenience a baby girl or a baby boy into a mother's infant.

We are faced here with a dogged prejudice: at the beginning, there are no parents with baby girls or boys, there are mothers and children whose sex is undifferentiated. And this implies that children who had everything (a penis) like boys or nothing (no penis) like girls, now become naughty, aggressive and sexually undifferentiated. One can note the transition here between the Freudian Oedipal theory which oscillates between 'one' (the internal problem of castration) and 'three' (the Oedipal trio) and the post-Freudian dual or object-relation theory (mother and child).

Considering the child firstly according to the penis' presence or absence, and secondly according to the mother-child couple, is coherent with a value judgment which haunts the whole history of mankind. We are confronted by some sort of fatality which leads women who lack the erect penis to be condemned to become mothers by the hearth, and men too scared at the idea of losing it to go to war. And the value judgment will generally favour men and disparage women or, as a reaction formation, favour mothers and disparage fathers. This is simply hopeless and totally discouraging.

To overcome this, we must urgently re-establish the balance between girls and boys. Penis or no penis, from the beginning girls and boys exist, and female genitals are different from male genitals, but neither worse nor better. Boys and girls are both subject to castration anxiety or castration belief - a fantasy shared with their parents. And the female characteristics should have the same value as the male's. Mothers and fathers can have children, boys or girls. That a mother gets pregnant and breast-feeds the infant, and that a man can have an erect penis are facts, not value judgments. Men and women are different and complementary.

Nowadays it seems that these wrongful representations of a devalued baby girl who has no tap, no pipe for micturition but who nevertheless urinates, an absence which is interpreted as an absence of a sexually invested penis, is outmoded, and the developing field of virtual reality with the use of the internet confirms this. As the female authors mentioned above maintain, females are fully equipped for a sexual life and have no reason whatsoever to envy the male's penis, nor, one might add, do males have any reason to envy females' vagina. Thus, from a biological as well as from a cultural perspective, men and women are genitally and sexually different but equal and psychoanalysts who agree with this statement (but who wouldn't agree?) should cease to overvalue the baby boy or devalue the baby girl and also to overvalue the mother and devalue the father.

Some analysts, still faithful to castration based on this invisible anatomic characteristic of the female sex, or to castration as a normally and constitutionally formed reaction to the missing penis, agree fully with feminine masochism: women suffer from lust for penetration, they are not jealous but envious, submissive and passive (passivity being considered morally as negative and activity as positive). Concomitantly, menstruation and menopause are equally considered a physiological loss which underlines once again the devalued characteristics of the woman - deprived of a penis - and does not take into consideration normal female characteristics without disparaging comparisons with the male. To confirm female castration using adult female physiological facts considered symbolically is, in my eyes, an attempt at retroprojection intended to validate so-called feminine masochism.

As far as I am concerned, I believe in the equal value of the sexes even if some women will consider me naïve. Surely, they would say, museums the world over would not be filled with Renaissance paintings of suffering virgin mothers with their baby boys, painted by men, if men had not known how to use their brushes and if women had not been content with their lot in life?

As we know, some prominent analysts have reacted to the castration complex and its devaluing aspects: the female sex organ is a container and corresponds to the need of the male sex organ to be contained, *i.e.* to penetrate. This could signify that there is no discrimination between sexes. Unfortunately this container mainly appears to have been filled up with children and the female has become the mother, who now is overvalourised vis-à-vis the male gender who in turn is devalourised and reduced to nothingness. So the container and its contents have been desexualised and transformed into a symbolic way of referring to the analyst and his analysand.

* * *

As an analyst, I shall add two observations in support of my thesis:

First, the analytic community seems to consider that men and women are equally qualified for their work. Obviously, their feelings and thinking are not the same, nor is their way of working. But the difference in gender does not matter. This does not mean that it is not taken into consideration. A patient might prefer an analyst of a particular gender; an analyst may feel more comfortable with a patient of this or that gender. But in the end, these preferences can be interpreted, and eventually cease to be significant. In 1920, Freud interrupted the analysis of a homosexual female patient. The study of his paper shows that his motivations were perfectly respectable but that he could have gone beyond them, had he become aware of the sore points aroused in him by his patient in the context of an Oedipal father/daughter transference relationship. I thus believe that a male analyst is no better or worse than a female or a mother analyst. This pleads in favour of a unique libido or sexual instinct which thrusts or seeks to satisfy the undesirable Oedipal desire. It is a refutation of the threat of castration for the boy and of its reality for the girl. A «real» baby girl lacking a penis of her own can be forgotten, it is a fantasy. Females are what they are. There is no devalourisation of a female's worth vis-à-vis a male's. Castration is an illusory virtual reality, a fantasy for both genders.

My second comment concerns the consequences of the baby girl castration theory: it is a female rebellion. The Kleinian rebellion in particular is spectacular. In short, the Kleinian female castrates the castrator. Sex is secondary, what counts is aggressiveness and the mother/child entity. Not the mother, the father's wife and her baby girl or baby boy, but the mother and the infant. This can be illustrated using a well-known Kleinian mechanism, projective identification. Klein negates (how right!) but/and projects her castrated baby-girl-self on Freud. He is castrated of his castration theory. And she becomes the psychoanalyst, the male. Then she denies the sexual problem and asserts herself as a mother without a husband, Freud being the naughty, sexually undifferentiated child. Eventually a compromise is reached through object-relationship. Freud is the psychoanalyst interested in sexuality according to his own sexuality and Klein is the psychoanalyst interested in the object-relation stemming from her relationship with Freud. But, unfortunately, not on an equal basis: for Kleinians a psychoanalyst is Kleinian or nothing. For Freudians a psychoanalyst does not need to be a Freudian analyst, simply an analyst. In so doing the Kleinian female deprives the Freudian male of his phallic privilege. But she also castrates herself of her sexual womanhood. She is the mother, the birth-giving mother. And her child, whatever its gender, is the aggressive child, destroyer of her breasts.

The Freudian castration complex is despair stemming from the past. It can never be overcome: the vision of the anatomy transforms the fantasy into a constituent of the psyche, a psychic structure.

The Kleinian mother/child entity is the making of despair. It can never be overcome; the depressive position is a sign of renunciation. One will never be one's own mother whatever one's efforts.

To overcome this deadlock, my thesis is that both the castration complex and the mother/child entity are fantasies, important and omnipresent fantasies in analysis, but without structure. For me, as an analyst, the fundamental structure of the psyche remains the Oedipal complex, this paramount Freudian discovery which helps to encompass narcissistic phenomena and object-relationship phenomena either dual or triangular.

In my opinion, the Oedipus complex is the structure or mode of the psychic apparatus from the analytical point of view, not that of a universal psyche, from the very psychic apparatus of the immature analysand and of his/her immature analyst. During analysis, both strive to satisfy and simultaneously rid themselves of their Oedipus complex, *i.e.* of the undesirable desire (the incestuous urge) which structures their relationship. And the question is: what are they finally aiming at? Maturity, I would reply, where the undesirable desire has been ousted.

In the analytical context, maturity appears as a transcendental ideal which can, from time to time, be perceived, felt through what I call «*la jouissance du dit* », (arousal and relief from what has been spoken aloud), when glimpses of true intersubjectivity allow each participant to recognise their partner as a subject in their own right and no longer as solely an object of desire.

## 4. A PERSONAL POINT OF VIEW

Yet the fact remains that the castration complex and the mother/child entity still lead to fruitful theoretical elaborations which illuminate innumerable and difficult clinical problems.

In order to keep the sexual differences and to avoid the devalourisation or overvalourisation of one of the two genders, an attitude which is prevalent outside our profession (and which has obviously no meaning whatsoever as far as dreams are concerned, these psycho-sexual windows on our unconscious), I propose that each gender be considered to be castrated of the gender it is not, of its embryological lost sex organ, loss of the parent whose gender is not the same as the child's. And consequently, each gender may dread losing its own. Castration fantasy is an illusory virtual reality. The rationalistic fiction of the threat fits the reality of the difference. There is no negation of the difference, but the imbalance in favour of boys is obsolete. The scale must be re-set to weigh what is thought to be «phallic»... or «castrated» taking into consideration the clinical difficulties arising from such a belief.

The threat of castration is a truth anchored in a lie. It stems from the shaky moral authority of the adult over the child and leads to super-ego formations, whatever the gender.

Here, we have to recognise the fact that infantile sexuality exists from the beginnings of life, that the adult is puzzled by it. The adult may be upset or even aroused when he or she sees manifestations of children's sexuality, however transient or superficial. And the consequence of this arousal is a loss of authority (Castel, 1998), an authority necessary for the child's upbringing. This is the source of castration (and not any anatomical lack): The adults negate their arousal and project it in a reverse way onto the child 'there is nothing to look at, stop it, or…'. Thus, they recover their authority. As a rule the threat leads to repression, the child's Oedipal desire will be concealed, reversed, *etc.*, in order to be preserved while by the same token satisfying and misleading the figure of authority. Repression finds its causal explanation in the sexual drive which provides energy for these distortions and its deep, unconscious meaning in the fact that sexuality endlessly entices the undesirable Oedipal urge, accompanied by a necessary token of submission to authority.

Castration, which rests on the illusory and deceitful threat of the adult seeking to impose his or her authority, can be understood as a virtual concept bound to the reality of a child's gender. It is a psychoanalytical virtual reality, a fantasy, a psychoanalytical truth. It has nothing to do with anatomy, with a boy's penis and a girl's clitoris.

The revival of Oedipal sexuality through interaction on the Internet, and considering castration to be a parental lie and a child's fantasy, lead to some fascinating new perspectives on psychoanalytical therapy.

Transsexuals, for instance, could experiment with their other gender through relationships on the computer screen, and evaluate whether the surgical mutilation they crave is really worthwhile and if not, choose instead to undertake analysis.

Anorexic girls could be seen as concealing under an oral symptomatology a terrifying anal fantasy of being sodomised by the father, a fantasy forged on the parental lie denying them a vagina and based on their Oedipal urge, with only the anus at their disposal for realisation. The little girl devoid of a penis, castrated, nevertheless has sexual interests and arousal (for instance when she lifts up her skirt, a blatant example indeed). Therefore, we may assume that the disapproving and castrating environment imposed on her by adults leads her to displace her sexual sensations onto the digestive apparatus which becomes sexually cathected and fellatio (described by Freud as a displacement and remnant from nursing) and sodomy become sexual substitutes for incestuous fantasies. Just as defaecation and faeces become disgusting and shameful in childhood, the sexual fantasies linked to the digestive apparatus become intolerable and may lead to anorexia. Of course this does not explain why a particular girl becomes anorexic, but it may give an interesting clue to understanding this terrible pathology and help the doctor with these difficult and demanding patients. One must realise that one's own words may be felt by the other to be an unbearably odious and perverse penetration.

As was the case for the dramatic outbreak of hysteric disorders which disappeared at the beginning of the past century, why couldn't we envision an end to this tragic pathology in the course of the 21$^{st}$ Century?

## 5. VERBAL ORGASM

If we consider the psychoanalytical experience in the light of a continuous thrust of the libido, which is necessary to perpetuating the undesirable Oedipal urge without which we cannot work, these entanglements between fantasy and facts should be corrected: how could a frightened male analyst, an envious female analyst or a non-maternal analyst work properly? They cannot. On the other side, intellectual endeavours and intelligence cannot be the attributes of male phallicism, and emotions and feelings that of feminine masochism.

My proposition of «*la jouissance du dit*» (arousal and relief coming from that which has been spoken aloud) aims at formulating these ideas as we hope to live them in analysis: enjoying thanks to libidinal cathexis, what is being said in the intersubjective conjuncture as something not undesirable, as the exciting and relieving discovery that our difficulties stem from the undesirable Oedipal urge and, once understood, that we may cease to endlessly pluck the same string.

«*La jouissance du dit*» could also be translated by 'verbal orgasm', an inadequate choice in my view because of its physiologic connotation. I would prefer 'verbal coming' in reference to the common use of the word during sexual intercourse. The crux of the matter is the turning point from transference to plain reality. Verbal arousal stemming from the dialogue with the Oedipus object turns into relief once this object appears as a subject. The arousal of the child (his or her highly undesirable desire towards his/her incestuous parent on the verge of being acted within or acted out) turns into relief thanks to the mutation and recognition of the object as a subject in its own right, a living human being, an analyst. At this point one becomes aware of the possibility of turning one's back on the past and looking to the future. Analysis ought to be based on hope, hope of overcoming this undesirable Oedipal urge, whatever the patient's gender.

The problem of outcome in analysis has always haunted psychoanalysts. One of the main difficulties arises when we consider it during analysis. It is almost impossible to avoid the dilemma between formation reaction and sublimation, two sides of the same coin. Is the ending of analysis an acting out? Obviously it is, from the point of view of the sessions: an acting out of the transference relationship. Is it something else? Yes, but in this case it can logically be considered only from the exterior or afterwards, once the relationship has ended. During analysis we cannot escape the Oedipal situation until the very end. But, on the other hand, external to analysis, in ordinary life, it may, surprisingly, appear perfectly similar to an analytical mind: Freud did show us that dreams - including his own - can always be interpreted in the light of the undesirable Oedipus desire - the incestuous urge - whatever the age or the skills. However old and experienced male or female analysts may get, such dreams and unconscious desires will follow them until death.

## 6. CONCLUSIONS

One could say that, from an analytical standpoint, we are all immature-psychically immature, whatever our age or intellectual achievements, however dignified, serious and respectable we appear; that we are always striving to satisfy the undesirable Oedipus desire. A puzzling deadlock indeed.

As previously mentioned, this means that the Oedipus complex builds, structures and organises our immature psychoanalytical personality (not the mundane, ordinary one), this very immaturity which transforms, alters the other or makes of him or her a thing, an object, the object of the undesirable desire. Once one has developed a taste for analysis, apparently it is for life.

The unconscious is an unknown language, the language of mankind's immaturity, a language which does not aim at other people, other selves, other subjects, but at objects of one's own self, things/objects we believe likely to satisfy the Oedipus desire. To be able to express this in analysis with our common, shared, day-to-day words, with our own bodily and mortal mother tongue which links us to our partner, analyst or analysand, leads us to perceive occasionally, to feel intuitively, to see this very partner in a flash or after some time not only as an object of our own but as a subject of his or her own. This is the arousal and relief through what has been spoken, an arousal bursting out from the presence of a living subject other than ourselves, a subject who is not our object. In analysis, we are both linked and separated through what is said, and once we have lived this true intersubjectivity, we may envision the ending of our unending quest for objects.

Maturity appears, therefore, as a transcendental ideal (inner but unreachable) and also a necessity to contemplate. Something to hope for in the future whatever it may be, gloomy or glorious, in order to end the analysis. Maturity does not mean anything more than the ability to renounce our fascination for the Oedipus desire in favour of an unknown future.

If the castration complex is no longer what it used to be, having expelled the concept of the devalourisation of the female anatomy through castration and the concomitant devalourisation of her psycho-sexuality, this of course does not signify the end of our difficulties. As soon as the dilemma generated by gender difference is overcome, the enjoyment of talking about it is juxtaposed to another analytical, anthropologically-based claim arising from the fact of death and its theoretical elaboration through the death instinct.

This could become understandable if we think of the object of the Oedipal wishes as immortal, a thing-object of ours, replaced by a living subject, a mortal being.

When confronted by an immortal object haunting their lives, people may develop death wishes towards it or towards themselves in order to escape the deadlock of their undesirable desire. Hence, the death instinct. Once the object is recognised as a mortal subject in his or her own right, death becomes part of life and does not require a special instinct. I surmise that the death instinct is a valid concept for those whose psychoanalytical mindset outweighs ordinary considerations. Object-relation oriented analysts belong to the first group; they are mainly concerned with the Oedipal or narcissistic dilemma and appreciate the death instinct as a realistic explanatory tool. Ego-psychology oriented analysts belong to the second; they are mainly oriented towards the elaboration of a self which is delivered of the Oedipal dilemma and does not need a theoretical fantasmatic death instinct. But, whatever the case, here again I believe that psychoanalysts cannot survive without a specific, analytical hope in our life time: the hope of discarding and overcoming the Oedipal desire by formulating it within psychoanalytical discourse, which, as I said, means the hope of re-directing our desire towards the unknowable future (my «*jouissance du dit*»).

Moral balance and male/female differences also lead to the hope of both genders participating equally in the destiny of the world. Should this be the case a Freudian utopia, a sea change in how society's institutions are run - the Church, the military, governments, *etc.* - becomes possible. The woman would no longer be condemned to the terrifyingly impotent, solitary, «good enough» mother role, guilty and responsible for the baby's destiny. The man would no longer be condemned to be the political, economic or religious, tyrannical leader. There is no need to exhibit a chest covered with medals - the rewards for the ability to destroy or kill.

Analysis is obviously a human science, a moral science and a life science while seeking an explanation for, and an understanding of the beginnings of life in order to improve the future. Psychoanalysis and the neurosciences, both life sciences, don't have to be antagonistic, they are complementary.

**References**

Ameisen, J.C. *La sculpture du vivant.* Editions du Seuil, Paris 1999

Castel, P.H. *Introduction à l'interprétation du rêve de Freud.* Presses Universitaires de France 1998

Odzer, Cleo *Sex and the cybercitizen.* Virtual spaces, Berkley books, New York 1997
Palac, Lisa *The edge of the bed.* Little, Brown and Company, 1998
Turkle, Sherry *Life on the screen.* Phoenix 1997

# From S. Freud to J. Bowlby: Infantile Sexuality; Is it Still a Scandalous Subject?

Bernard Golse
*Professor of Psychiatry de l'Hopital St Vincent de Paul, Paris*

## 1. THE SEDUCTION THEORY

I would first of all like to recall that this year we are celebrating the hundredth anniversary of S. Freud's renunciation of his neurotica (Letter 69 to W. Fliess of 21st September 1897) which, as we know, opened the path to the etiological theory of imaginary trauma, in opposition to that of real trauma.

A hundred years on, infantile sexuality is still, in my opinion, a scandalous topic. Resistance to its recognition has taken on the mask of pseudo-liberalism and banality.

The way the topic is presented today basically says: «All this is common knowledge, S. Freud talked about it a long time ago, so there's no need to weigh in on the subject... ». And so the hand is played: infantile sexuality retires from the stage, taking with it its most profound functions and significance.

However, as we know, there is no repression without consequences... and we need only check out today's headlines to gauge the media attention given to crimes of paedophilia.

Of course, the children who are victims of these crimes deserve all our attention and care so that their psychic future does not remain heavily scarred by these dramatic occurrences. But what I want to say is that interest in the real trauma of children should in no way serve as an alibi to massively evacuate the perspective of imaginary traumatism and infantile sexuality in all its aspects.

To understand trauma effectively requires taking into account its dual reality - internal and fantasmatical on the one side, external and factual history on the other, and it is only thus that the effectiveness of the trauma can be seen to be usefully perceived (J. Laplanche).

# 2. THE EVOLUTION OF IDEAS

## 2.1 First Remark

The passage from an orificial psychoanalysis, especially one focusing on content and the traumatisms resulting from excess or intrusion, to a more skin-deep psychoanalysis focused on containers (psychic envelopes) and hollow traumatisms which lack a container (a negative or void clinical aspect), is one which, it seems to me, has occurred progressively over the second half of the $20^{th}$ century, bearing witness notably to the intense current interest for maternal depression. This passage carries the risk of a certain surreptitious desexualisation of the psychoanalytical body.

The question of classical partial erogenous zones and therefore of drives is indeed somewhat diluted and A. Green rightly reminds us to be careful to avoid echoing ourselves the dangers we stress in our conceptual environment.

## 2.2 Second Remark

We reproached S. Freud for having given a slightly over-solipsistic vision to psychoaffective and sexual development in the child - which moreover, an attentive reading of his work as a whole would probably disprove.

Nonetheless, his successors have no doubt accentuated the importance of the interrelation and weight of unconscious fantasmatic parental dynamics in the gradual structuring of the child's psyche.

In this perspective, both D.W. Winnicott and W.R. Bion insist on the detour through the other which has proved to be necessary in setting up the psychic apparatus of the child. Again, A. Green, indicated this clearly by grouping those who shared this view, as opposed to S. Freud and M. Klein who focused far more on the dynamics which come into play for the child and less on the adult/child couple such as it is.

In any case, we can no longer speak of the psychic development of the child outside the relationship, an apprehension which, according to J. Laplanche, would simply end up in a veritable 'desert island' situation.

In other words, to establish and test one's self as such, the psychic apparatus must first allow itself to think of another psyche (A. Green, 1990), the dynamics of ontogenesis are thus found, mutatis mutandis, in those of the treatment.

Indeed, this interactive or interrelational vision of the growth and psychic maturity of the child invites us, regardless of context, to accord a place of honour to infantile sexuality, that of the child and the adult who was once a child, as well as that of the child itself, all of which are inextricably linked and inevitably interwoven...scandalously so!

## 3. DEVELOPMENT AND DESTINY

Putting these two ideas into perspective sheds light on the place occupied by infantile sexuality through the effects of encounter as was so well shown by C. Bollas, in «The Forces of Destiny», positioning himself as he did in relation to the double heritage of S. Freud and D.W. Winnicott.

As we know, S. Freud was in some ways more destiny- than development-oriented. In the «Three Essays on the Theory of Sexuality», his chapter on drives is in fact entitled «Drives and their Destiny» and not «Drives and their Development».

This dispels any lingering doubts by underlining the fact that S. Freud did not have a purely biological vision of psychosexual development, as programmed and endogenous, but a very mixed, endogenous and exogenous vision, an interface between the biological and the relational. For Freud, nevertheless, fate is not destiny, as discussed in the work of C. Bollas in reference to D.W. Winnicott's concepts of truth and the false self.

Indeed, for C. Bollas, the idea of destiny can be used to define the feeling a person can have in relation to their life story, that their true self has not been fulfilled, or facilitated by life experience.

The idea of destiny can thus be thought of as referring back to the concept of the «false self» whereas that of destiny should refer back to the evolution of the «true self». It is thus destiny, in its more or less harmful fatalistic dimension, which threatens to cause us to elude our destiny, to stop us from fulfilling it. The destiny drive would then represent the force of «the idiom» of the subject which tends towards the constitution of the true self, at the very crossroads of the endogenous potentialities of the individual and the different encounters made or missed in regard to objects, the effect of an encounter which simultaneously includes the way these objects will be used, and the way in which the individual will succeed or fail in utilising these objects (starting with the mother, notably her ability to be separate).

Without wishing to confuse matters further, I am willing to say that fate, in the definition given to it by C. Bollas, corresponds somewhat to fate as seen by the Ancient Greeks for whom justice could only be obtained by a given individual if he was able to accomplish his true destiny, during his lifetime.

However, the difference lies in the fact that C. Bollas' notion of destiny is founded on an immanent, true self which is intrinsically human, whereas fate in Greek Antiquity is founded on a horizon assigned by divine intervention which is extrinsic to the individual who it transcends.

However each of these cases, in my view appear to contain the idea of appropriateness to the profound potentiality of the subject.

In favourable cases, fate and destiny can be interchangeable. In unfavourable cases, fate hampers us from fulfilling our destiny. This strikes a chord in me when I think of the children we treat and their futures.

In any case, therein lies the foundation of a dialectic between the internal and external worlds as far as the growth and psychic maturity in the child are concerned, if we must avoid the word development on all accounts.

Finally, this provides an authentic place for infantile sexuality, since the encounter with the object, regardless of questions of acceptance or shock or whether this is played out against a background of fascination or of terror can never be conceived in its inevitable atmosphere of seduction.

## 4. FROM S. FREUD TO J. BOWLBY: ATTACHMENT AS A PARADIGM SUSCEPTIBLE TO LINK THE THEORY OF DRIVES AND THE THEORY OF RELATIONS WITH THE OBJECT

It is not a question of being ecumenical at all costs, but simply of being honest. While some might conceive or use the theory of attachment partly at least to evacuate the scandal of infantile sexuality, in reality this theory does not appear to impose the revisions which some have referred to as ripping metapsychology apart. This is what I tried to show in the article published in the *Monographies de Psychopathologie,* entitled: «Attachment, working internal models and metapsychology, or how not to throw the baby out with the bathwater?» If the attachment corresponds to a primary need in the child, why not imagine that it can be libidinalised like all other needs in the theory of anaclisis?

In any case, this attachment cannot, in my view be conceptualised in purely cognitive terms. Even in the «Strange Situation» of M. Ainsworth, different types of attachment of the baby are described in terms of affect (secure attachment, insecure or anxious attachments, avoidant attachment...)

and the schematics of attachment should be considered as a mixture of the cognitive and the affective. In other terms, the object of attachment is simultaneously found to be an object to be discovered and an object of investment.

The working internal models described by J. Bowlby, M. Main and I. Bretherton notably bear the status of mental representations, perceived after J. Bowlby's death in 1990, as being less absent from his theory than we might have supposed.

The work of M. Main on Adult Attachment Interview (A.A.I.), which was taken over by the team of B. Pierrehumbert in Lausanne, clearly shows that the fantasmatical transgenerational transmission of patterns of attachment follows the mechanisms of fantasmatical transmission as much as those of cognitive transmission whose heritage is more or less genetic.

I would add that all this research on attachment undeniably leaves room for the after-effect. P. Fonagy, for example (of the Anna Freud Centre in London), has shown that very strong correlations exist, approximately 80%, between the type of response of the mother to A.A.I. and the nature of the patterns of attachment of the baby evaluated in the «Strange Situation». In other words, a mother whose hindsight, rightly or wrongly, shows security or insecurity in her own links of attachment, will, in almost 80% of cases, induce attachment patterns in her child which are respectively secure or insecure.

However, A.A.I. gives access to current representations that the adult creates for him- or herself of early procedures of attachment and these representations are obviously found to be re-mixed and re-constructed out of a whole series of distortions and intermediate repression.

This suggests that the birth and the interactive presence of the baby reactivate the mother's past experiences of early childhood, through an after-effect, notably in the field of attachment. These past experiences will then infiltrate the qualitative nature of the system of relationships the mother subsequently presents to her child.

The setting up, finally, of attachment patterns by the baby is played out by what D.N. Stern calls the «representations of generalised interaction» at the heart of which absence, difference and distance occupy an essential place.

The child effectively extracts from his or her different interactive experiences a means, or fictitious result never experienced as such but written into the psyche of the child as an abstraction of the interactive style of his or her principal partners in relationships, if we wish to understand an activity of extraction of invariables in terms of abstraction.

During each effective interactive encounter in reality, the child will in some ways measure the gap between what he or she experiences at the instant and this dynamic and prototypical representation he or she has created of the adult, a difference which informs him or her about the adult's emotional state (affective agreement or harmonisation of affects).

In my view, taking account of the theory of attachment does not mean we have to in any way renounce metapsychology - and therefore infantile sexuality - particularly as the separation referred to above serves in some ways as «a bed of third parties».

## 5. SUMMARY

The introduction of attachment theory gave rise to well-publicised polemics. It caused a number of psychoanalysts to undergo a harrowing re-examination of metapsychology leading many to relinquish the theory of drives, the theory of the dimensions of impact of the sexual drive and the theory of deferred action, short-circuiting the question of mental representations and giving priority to the presence of the object rather than the impact of its loss, its absence or its exclusion.

In fact, the whole issue of infantile sexuality has been raised by this trend in beliefs. We would like to show that, while collective resistance to psychoanalysis has certainly adopted the attachment theory to try to get rid of the concept of infantile sexuality, the attachment theory actually in no way excludes it, if we conceive of attachment as a possible bridge between the theory of drives and the theory of object relations.

It is in this perspective that it may be possible for us to restore infantile sexuality to its rightful place in all its aspects, without sensationalising media headlines or serving financial interests linked to extreme cases (ill-treatment, sexual abuse..). Although these certainly deserve our attention, they may sometimes distract us from a more profound understanding of the trauma in both its realistic and imaginary aspects.

Infantile sexuality is a scandalous concept, as it was in the past and will continue to be, but the forms that resistance takes - whether individual, theoretical or social - have probably changed and are creating obstacles to a better understanding of the true nature of its current impact.

# New Psychoanalytic Views on Bisexuality

Didier Houzel
*French Psychoanalytical Association*

## 1. CONCEPT

The concept of psychic bisexuality appeared early in the history of psychoanalysis (in Freud's letter to Fliess dated 6th December 1896), and undoubtedly played a role in the discovery and description of the Oedipus complex in both its positive and negative aspects. But it has not, perhaps, been allowed to give its full measure, in particular in the analysis of pre-Oedipal development and the working of the mind in this early period. It is true, of course, that Melanie Klein's description of the early stages of the Oedipus conflict constituted a decisive step in the exploration of the early phases of psychic bisexuality. I feel, however, that a further step remains to be taken - that of examining the relevance of the idea of psychic bisexuality at the most primitive levels of the origins of the mind and the deep-seated strata of the psychic apparatus, as Tustin suggested. These are the configurations which lie at the root of narcissism and support individuation, and they correspond to what W.R. Bion called the container, Bick the psychic *skin* and D, Anzieu first the *skin-ego* then the *psychic envelope*, this implies that we consider three levels where psychic bisexuality is involved and where the problem of integrating masculine and feminine aspects arises- first, the *psychic envelope,* then *part-object relations*, and, finally, *whole object relations.*

To each of these levels corresponds a pattern of integration of bisexuality, in which the maternal or feminine aspects and the paternal or masculine ones can come together in a complementary and balanced manner.

## 2. THE BISEXUALITY OF THE PSYCHIC ENVELOPE

The psychic envelope has the care-giving aspects of the mother as its principal foundation. Nevertheless, the quality of the relationship between mother and infant depends, on the one hand, on the quality of her own bisexual identifications, paternal as well as maternal, and on the other, on the support she receives from her immediate environment, most noticeably that of her husband. It is as though, in order to function adequately, the maternal elements have to be reinforced by paternal aspects if the psychic envelope is to have the necessary qualities. It is only if this criterion is satisfied that the psychic envelope will have resiliency and elasticity. It must be receptive, extensible and yielding, so that the infant can leave its mark on it. This corresponds to the form of primitive communication that Klein called *projective identification*, and that Bion declared to be the original form of communication from mind to mind. But the psychic envelope must also be solid and resistant, so that it will neither be knocked out of shape nor punctured. I place its receptive, extensible and yielding qualities on the side of the maternal or feminine aspects, and its solidity and resistance on the paternal or masculine side. When these different features are adequately integrated, the psychic envelope will have the necessary degree of elasticity.

To my mind, the psychoanalytic exploration of autism and early infantile psychoses involves consideration of the differences between feminine and masculine from a somewhat different angle, for what we are faced with in such syndromes is a pathology of otherness. The question of individuation corresponds, in my view, to the problem of integrating bisexuality within the psychic envelope. To be able to differentiate oneself from other people, to establish a frontier between Self and Object, to tolerate separateness from the other with all it implies in terms of distance, limits, differences and frustrations - this is the issue involved in any relationship with a container (or envelope) endowed with bisexual qualities combined in the correct proportions.

To my way of thinking, it is very important to recognise that it is the same containing object which must possess feminine/maternal and masculine/paternal features in the correct proportions. It is not possible, at such an early developmental stage, to differentiate between a maternal part- or whole object and a paternal one. The fact has to be acknowledged that there are some paternal features in the maternal containing object. Any paternal element which is dissociated from the container will be experienced as threatening, persecutory and destructive. This is probably what occurs in the autistic child, who very early in life splits off the component parts of psychic bisexuality, probably because he is at that stage unable to find enough paternal features in his mother. I refer here specifically to two masculine components of the containers' bisexuality - the mother's own paternal identifications, and the support she receives from her husband, the child's father or surrogate father. On this point, it is interesting to note that in a study of the factors predictive of the quality of the father-child relationship, Feldman *et al.* found that the quality of the mother's relationship with her own father was a crucial factor. The masculine/ paternal aspects of the mother seem to prepare the way for the father, in a kind of invitation to acknowledge the father's place. If this does not happen, it seems impossible for the father to take up his rightful place in the child's psychic economy and to play a structuring role in its personality development.

In therapy, it is mainly by working through the counter-transference that the psychoanalyst can help the child reintegrate split-off parts of psychic *bisexuality* in the containing object. Tustin stressed time and again how important it is, in conducting psychotherapy, to exhibit not only a great deal of responsiveness and receptivity, but also a certain degree of firmness - another instance of the maternal/feminine and paternal/masculine duality of the containing function. In my view, what Anne Alvarez calls «live company» and her idea of the reclaiming function refer also to the need to integrate paternal elements into the maternal containing function (the analyst's attentive listening).

As I mentioned earlier, Tustin drew our attention to the deep splitting autistic children operate between these features of the psychic envelope, and to the way in which it is evidenced in terms of contrasting sensory qualities: dry/wet, rough/smooth, hard/soft, hot/cold, *etc.* Tustin related these split-off sensory attributes to a splitting of psychic bisexuality in the original container, describing how the autistic child seems to feel that the reunion of paternal/masculine and maternal/feminine qualities is a destructive and catastrophic experience. The factors Tustin identified in autistic children can also be found at the deepest levels of mental functioning in child and adult patients who present pathological states which, though they may be much less primitive, have nonetheless developed on the basis of an autistic enclave.

In my view, the maternal/feminine aspects of the container involve the flexible, yielding breast the baby enjoys toying vigorously with as it feeds, as though trying to impress on it the intense emotions this extraordinary experience arouses in it. The masculine/paternal aspects of the container would, in this view, relate to the nipple, the firm and erectile part of the combined nipple-and-breast object, standing guard between the baby's greedy mouth and the breast, protecting the latter against any attempt at destructive breaking and entering.

## 3. A CLINICAL ILLUSTRATION

1 would like to illustrate this topic with material taken from the analysis of one of my patients, an autistic boy. The session I shall narrate occurred after six years of therapy, at a rhythm of four sessions per week. Alain has made considerable headway during these six years of analysis; his speech has improved beyond all recognition; he attends school - in fact he has come through the whole of his primary schooling with only one year having to be repeated. He has made good progress in sociability; he takes part in games with other children, and his everyday behaviour is relatively well-adjusted. He does, however, quite often remain isolated, has many odd quirks and he frequently chatters on about things which bear no apparent relation to the external situation at any given time.

By the time this session took place, his speech was beginning to be more connected and he was narrating memories from the more or less distant past, some, in fact, from very early on in life. It is when they begin to emerge from their autistic state that such children are able to represent and to put into words the mental states, the pain and the fantasies that have been buried deep inside them from the earliest days of life.

I will distinguish between three sequences in this session: the first one describes an uncontaining maternal object, the second one the deflection onto the paternal object of uncontained and untransformed elements, and the third one the restoration of the containing function by integrating bisexuality.

### 3.1 An Uncontaining Maternal Object

Alain reminded me of the time in his analysis when he wanted to spit at me and I forbade him to do so. On one occasion, I had even threatened to interrupt the session if he did not stop. He questioned me at some length about what would have happened had the session indeed been interrupted. Would the taxi in which he came to his sessions have taken him back home? Would he have had to wait in the waiting-room?

He then went on to recall various circumstances in which sessions had been cancelled, and spoke of a forthcoming session that he knew I would be unable to maintain. What did I do during these missed sessions? Did I have a meeting? When he had been unable to come to his session, did I wait for him or did I just go home? In this way, Alain recalled a whole series of circumstances in which we had not met as planned.

Then he spoke of church bells falling silent on Good Friday because, as he put it, people are saddened by the death of Jesus; the bells come back on Easter Sunday because Jesus is resuscitated. He then attempted to tickle me, saying that it would be like the rotating lights at fun-fairs.

I replied that we were indeed sad every time we were apart, because of missed sessions or the holiday period which had just ended, sad like at the death of Jesus; but afterwards we were happy when we were together again, and then it was as though bells were ringing and rotating lights flashing. Alain went on to speak of things he called «disgusting» and «not polite». One day he had smelt Aunt Marie-Laure's armpits and his mother had smacked him. Another time, he had demanded a biscuit and his mother had scolded him. He told me about a pony that had diarrhoea. Alain had made what he called «pony-droppings» by soaking paper in water and rolling it into little balls, then he had thrown them at the walls of his room.

At that point I recalled something his parents had told me. When the family had gone to live abroad (for reasons to do with the father's work), Alain had suffered from severe diarrhoea which, resisting all attempts at medication, had lasted several months. He was 9 months old at the time. His previous development had in any case been abnormal: he seldom smiled, he screamed a lot, and his parents were concerned even then about his difficulty in relating to others. The move abroad had intensified both his suffering and his withdrawal.

I said to Alain that what he was doing and saying reminded me of what his parents had told me - that when he was just a little baby, he had suffered from very severe diarrhoea which had gone on for a very long time. I added that he was perhaps wondering now whether I would be like a mummy who felt that what came out of him was disgusting (diarrhoea or «impoliteness»), or one who, on the contrary, would be able to accept all that kind of thing.

## 3.2 Deflection on to the Paternal Object of Uncontained and Untransformed Elements Impossible to Integrate

Alain went on to talk of the smell from people's armpits, a theme which is often on his mind. He sniffs at his father's armpits, and says they smell like leeks. I completed my interpretation with the statement that when he was very young he had gone to stay in a country where the climate was very hot; he had sweated a lot there, which no doubt, gave off a bad smell. I added that, in telling me of his father's armpits, maybe he was projecting everything bad onto his father in order to avoid having a mother who might reject him because of all the disgusting things that give off bad smells.

## 3.3 Restoring the Bisexuality of the Containing Object

Alain, who normally is very restless, became very calm at this, and began to tell me in some detail of a memory from his early childhood. He was going for a sail with his maternal grandfather, whom he calls Granpappy, in the latter's boat. He was 2 ½ years old at the time. He had felt sick, and had vomited about ten yards after the boat had sailed round a sonar buoy, which Alain described as a buoy with a bell. He told me how his mother had been annoyed at his vomiting and had scolded him. He described also how his grandfather had manoeuvred the boat so as to steer clear of some dangerous rocks.

I said he wanted me to be a mummy who would accept everything that came out of him, without finding it disgusting, a mummy who wouldn't get annoyed, a mummy who would be helped by a Granpappy manoeuvring to avoid danger.

The session I have narrated provides us with an illustration of what is at issue in the integration of bisexuality at its most primitive level, that of the original *container*. The containing function of the analysis is represented by the grandfather's sailing boat. Alain's recollection (screen-memory) reveals both the failures of the maternal container and the hope of repairing them by the use of the grandfather image to support the maternal function. Granpappy manoeuvring the boat-container in order to prevent its dashing against the rocks. This memory therefore indicates Alain's capacity to integrate psychic bisexuality in order to weave a containing envelope; it is this capacity which brings peace and tranquillity to him.

Every separation and every lapse in the rhythm of the sessions were, up till that point, felt by Alain to be failures in the *containing* function. The analytical setting seemed to be unable to take in and transform the boy's violent projections, as represented by his spitting, diarrhoea, vomiting and impoliteness. I agree with Anzieu when he claims that the psychic envelope is deposited onto the analytical setting and is not static in the way suggested by Bleger, for whom «conglomerated nuclei» are simply «deposited» onto the setting, but something very much more dynamic, resulting in attacks on the setting, the meaning of which, generally speaking, can only be made clear by working through the counter-transference.

# 4. BISEXUALITY IN PART-OBJECT RELATIONS

As soon as a psychic envelope is constituted, the distinction between interior and exterior becomes meaningful. From then on, the infant can introject objects into an inner mental space. We are now at the second level, that of part-object relations.

The part-object relation is characterised by a quest for certain qualities that are not only physical and sensory, but also psychic. In this case too, such qualities can be classified according to their feminine or masculine polarity. On the maternal/feminine side we have receptivity, tolerance, comfort and availability; while on the paternal/masculine side we find strength, solidity, coherence and a sense of direction. My aim is not, of course, to infer some kind of gender typology or an inflexible distribution of these psychic qualities as between man and woman. Both sexes have bisexual features that must coexist and balance each other out, though perhaps in varying proportions.

I would suggest that the integration of psychic bisexuality on the part-object level is necessary if the process of stabilising the internal world is to succeed. Two types of link contribute to this stabilisation. The first, which I shall call, the «nipple-link» sets up the relationship between the self and the nourishing maternal object, the «nourishing breast» as Klein put it; it is a proximal link. The second, the "penis-link", is distal, and sets up a relationship between self and object, whatever the gaps, distances or differences that lie between them. In the internal world, the question is one of differentiating between psychic areas as described by D. Meltzer, in order to acquire an axis and psychic verticality, with, in constructing the body image, symmetry between left and right and asymmetry between top and bottom. In the external world, the issue is one of establishing relationships with other objects, whatever the discontinuities caused by frustration, the distances created by absence, and other types of difference: between self and other (otherness), between genders, between generations.

These two types of link are characterised both by continuity and by major transformations. The nipple-link is the heir to the masculine/paternal aspect of the primary containing object and prepares the way for the penis-link. A complex process of differentiation is required in order to sort out these two types of link, which are often mixed up - particularly in the perversions.

## 5. BISEXUALITY AND WHOLE-OBJECT RELATIONS

Now the context becomes that of the Oedipus conflict as described by Freud. Integration of bisexuality at this third level is the process which leads to the establishment of sexual identity. From the point of view of the mind, we become man or woman by identifying with the parent of the same sex. This cannot, however, be an inflexible identification that leaves no room for cross-identification with the parent of the opposite sex - it is on the equilibrium between these two identifications that the stability of sexual identity depends.

I do not intend to repeat the well-known description of the positive and negative Oedipus complex. I must, nonetheless, insist on one aspect of psychic bisexuality at this level of integration, since it involves what I would call mediation of one parental object by the other. We have known for some time now how important it is for the infant's relationship to the mother to be mediated by the father; the barrier against incest, with its links to the paternal superego, is a commonly-acknowledged expression of this mediation. Reparation, which Klein associated with paternal identification, is another aspect of this. The father is not the «great separator» as Lacan claimed him to be, rather he is a kind of binding force that determines a relationship with the mother which is neither engulfing nor destructive. At the same time, the maternal object is there, in my view, to mediate the paternal one; without such mediation, the father would be no more than a threat, a castrator and a persecutor. He would resemble the statue of the commander in Molière's Don Juan, suddenly and brutally demanding an explanation of past wrong-doing, and leaving no room for redemption: Don Juan is thrown into hell. When there is no mediation of one parental object by the other, extremism dominates.

## 6. CONCLUSIONS

As we reach the end of this discussion, I would like to make one more brief remark. The advent of the Oedipus conflict can be considered from two different points of view. The first - and in my opinion the dominant approach, at least in France - consists in assuming that there is an initial phase in life during which the mother-baby relationship is exclusive of all others, *i.e.* nothing paternal can intervene to disturb the infant's idyllic relationship with his constantly available and loving mother; it is only in due course that the father appears on the scene and interrupts the mother-baby duality, in order to demand his due and claim back his rightful place.

The second manner in which the Oedipus situation can be approached is to assume that there is a bisexual pattern in operation from the very outset, without which no relationship and no mental life can ever be possible. The pattern itself changes as the infant grows and its mental development continues.

To my way of thinking, the first of these approaches is too linear. It cannot give an adequate account of the processes that govern mental growth and its early pathological vicissitudes, in particular those encountered in infantile autism and the psychoses of childhood. I feel it much more satisfying to posit that there is a kind of psychic bisexuality in operation *ab initio*, from the very beginnings of extra-uterine life, the transformations which this psychic bisexuality undergoes are what confront us at different stages in development and in the various psychopathological states.

# Psychosexuality and Borderline Disorders

Alicia Schteingart-Gitnacht
*Swiss Psychoanalytical Society*

I will not address, in this paper, the factual history of the sexuality of borderline patients. However, if we begin by scratching the surface, by what is seen and acted upon, I will say that their behaviour is often surprising and does not pass unnoticed. Their audience is captivated by the fact that they wear their narcissism on their sleeve, narcissistically compelled to seduce, once seduction has been consummated, they become fickle, pulling the rug out from under the relationship: repudiating the object as soon as it feels loved, seeking it out again, once the object becomes convinced he or she has been rejected. I shall then address the internal, intrapsychic shifts which motivate this type of behaviour.

## 1. THE SEXUALITY OF BORDERLINES

Their sexual appetites vary greatly. They cover a wide spectrum: from the anorexic who won't eat, who physically exercises exhaustively and refuses any long-term relationship which might threaten sovereignty over his or her own body and over the object, with an enormous and astonishing greed which is never satisfied and which consumes objects like they were cocktail peanuts, as one patient told me. This attitude can be accompanied by a very intense sexuality. Bisexuality is common, interaction with reality is variable. As the object is very frustrating, the borderline has a tendency to change objects; he or she runs the gamut from the most desperate narcissism to a frenetic search for the object. Also, promiscuity often enters into the picture, as the continual search for satisfaction allows the patient to calm latent anxiety, aggressiveness and disorganisation.

Thus, at the same time as a patient sought to provoke me into a maternal, sado-masochistic - mainly sadistic - transference, she began to act out multiple sexual relationships, individual and group, homo- and heterosexual, which sprung from various causes, among them a lack of repression and a great difficulty in accepting frustration. Subsequently, we were able to understand how she attacked her parents' couple, using me as an intermediary. In this way, through transference she replicated her desire to humiliate her mother, to make her jealous and envious, to make her grovel at her feet: for example, the mother cleaned the shoes that the patient took pains to soil. This behaviour increased after seeing me in a shop with my husband one day. She also spoke to me about her ex-analyst, a man, and she explained how perfect and competent he was, an exact replica of her father. This might bring to mind an Oedipal rivalry, but this is grafted onto constant acting in and out and provocations that made the working-through process difficult. The aim of this process was essentially to create a psychic void. If I give this example, it is because it allows us to understand much more destructive situations. For this patient, structuring was enabled through sado-masochism. At superficial layers, it resembles hysteria. Other cases combine genital and pre-genital sexuality of all types. Perverse aspects may appear through homo- and heterosexual fantasies, fetishes and even paedophilia, sometimes latent, sometimes acted out.

## 2. METAPSYCHOLOGICAL POINT OF VIEW

I will now try to describe this type of patient at a more metapsychological level, which implies a set of examples coming from the first topographic point of view (conscious, preconscious, unconscious) and the second (ego, id, superego). I will add, to clarify comprehension, that borderline disorder, as the name suggests, involves difficulties with boundaries, those elements of the first topographic point of view not coinciding completely with those of the second. In addition, I consider that the points of fixation are important (orality, anality, phallicity), as well as the regression to these.

The relationship with the object is structured or twisted from the first exchanges with the mother. The degree of satisfaction or dissatisfaction is very important for the constitution of the early ego. The infant is built up out of the shift between satisfaction and frustration. The latter is just as important, as the mind is created out of alternating currents. A «good enough mother» has the capacity to dream, which fosters the ability in the infant to imagine the mother dreaming of him or her, but this mother is also capable of letting the infant cry, first from hunger and later from other needs. This creates a hallucinatory ability in the infant, according to Freud, which is the forebear of the ability to think thoughts. Through the intermediary of the function of the father, which cannot be forgotten as it provides organisation and separation, exchanges with the mother firstly promote the creation of a boundary. We call this boundary a «protective shield». From the symbiosis between mother and child, we can now pass on to the internal world of the child. Internal reality is not a reproduction of external reality. Children who have lived in situations of great neglect or frustration may sometimes have a highly structured psyche, which implies a capacity to love the object and keep it inside one's self. Other children, in contrast, may, despite apparently privileged circumstances, build their characters in a narcissistic fashion, which is negative and destructive. This is coupled, undoubtedly, according to what I have observed in analysis, with a high degree of parental permissiveness and a lack of clear limits. Which leads me to believe that, for certain patients, a good spanking given at the right time, might have done a world of good. I am thinking of a particular patient in analysis and of others too, whose inexplicable provocation was present at first encounter, and led to a narcissistic crisis and arguments during the session which resembled domestic squabbles. Their objective, even if the patient is not aware of it, is to provoke a fight or to get a symbolic spanking from the analyst in order to put an end to their destructiveness. Attacks on the real object in childhood, fantasised about subsequently and reproduced in transferential regression are often acted upon. Repetition may allow the setting up of symbolic links or prevent it. What I have just pointed out constitutes an element of prognosis of the highest importance. If the object, the analyst in transference, succeeds in staking his or her ground and in recreating the past and modifying it, he or she will already have made considerable gains. The patient who is unmanageable in any relationship and only comes to the analysis to relive the destructive cycle without being able to modify it, has a poor prognosis. This depends neither on the conscious will of the analyst nor, unfortunately, on that of the patient. It is from the encounter itself and its repercussions that we can, *a posteriori*, evaluate the ability of the patient to make a link, to profit from a relationship and to introject it. A very destructive patient will evacuate rather than incorporate, resulting in emotional and mental impoverishment, often bordering on deficiency. Another patient, in similar circumstances, will have a profitable encounter and will end up by introjecting a good relationship and thus manage to modify his or her object relations.

## 3. STRUCTURAL APPROACH

I would like to speak at present about the structure of borderline disorders, or rather of a scale of structures.

In my report to the French-Language Congress in 1998, I presented my point of view concerning anality. On this topic, I underline that in the anal expulsive stage (Stage I), the object is not considered as having already separated from the subject, it is expulsed without any consideration, soiled, mixed-up, destroyed. The object is not safeguarded, it is a question of its equalisation and its faecalisation. As sadism is primitive and imbued with a death wish, the re-introjection or the lack of projection of this kind of partial relationship destroys the subject at a mental or a physical level. In my view, these archaic mechanisms touch on the profound structure of the ego of the patient. When the ability to master the ego of the subject is threatened (because the issues of sovereignty and boundaries arising in the 2nd anal stage are scarcely present), dissociative mechanisms increase in intensity and in sadism. Wounded in their narcissism, they are often persecuted because of massive projective identification, and the renewal of conflict, which renders internal persecution «real». Their acting out of replays deforms primitive situations and they use their audience in such a way that the audience retaliates, knocking their projections back on to them, confirming the persecution mechanism. It is difficult to remain neutral and to function as an effective gatekeeper, as the analyst often comes under attack. In addition, when we act out of sympathy for their suffering and try to help them, they distort our intervention, transforming it into projection. We are sucked into a strange world where the rules of neurosis no longer apply. In the best of cases, perverse mechanisms organise their functioning.

## 4. CLINICAL EXAMPLE

To illustrate my theoretical assertions, I will discuss a borderline patient about whom I have spoken on other occasions. I will only say here that she came to me because she was suffering from Crohn's disease, displaying in addition a borderline functioning which oscillated between despair at the idea of solitude, mistreatment of the object, and persecution of the body. Another defence mechanism, manic and all-powerful, pushed her to scale mountain-tops, where her sovereignty over body and heights, sometimes in dangerous situations, allowed her, on one hand, to calm herself (an auto-calming mechanism as the Paris psychosomatic analysts would say) and, on the other, to feel like «an eagle flying over our heads» (manic mechanism). Nevertheless, as soon as she came back down to earth, the feeling of abandonment and despair took control again. When she could seduce, her attitude was also manic, triumphant. As she pled poverty, the physician she consulted for her intestinal complaint literally bought her food. The most stable relationship she conducted with a man during analysis was linked to the oral (he was obese) and maternal structure provided by her partner. Here she could recreate the mother-child relationship. She also seduced a much older professional who made her read philosophy. After having bragged about his qualities, she declared that he was boring and impotent and they had a falling out. Her associations at this period centred on fantasies of persecution of the body, linked first of all to her faeces and then to spermatozoa. «It's disgusting», she said «they invade my body and deform it». In contrast, she advocated homosexuality: «How exquisite are relationships between women!» Let us not forget that she provokes me in order to better seduce me. When sexual penetration in her relationship became unavoidable, she felt threatened, and expulsive mechanisms took over. This anxiety was manifested as much at the level of sexuality as that of object relations. In this instance, my word was used as an object that must be discarded if sovereignty were to be maintained. Penetration threatens sovereignty.

At present I will give a short clinical vignette.

She spoke of an episode which took place before her summer holidays, in the midst of innumerable aggravations. She began by complaining about her girlfriends, who have no manners, as they are rich and refined and don't want anything to do with her. In addition, X, whom I knew well, ignored her.

In order to make the story more lucid, I will say that the person in question was a young lady in my entourage of whom she is particularly jealous and envious. She felt love/hate/passion.

The following session brought some clarification. The girls were camping in a tent, they were gossiping and enjoying themselves. As she felt excluded, she began farting, something which was not at all appreciated. At least now she was excluded for a good reason and got revenge at the same time!

This anal behaviour is frequent in young children in therapy. It is the sign of an anal eroticism which is inseparable from sadism, at an archaic level. In this regression, which implies a fixation, gas, faecal matter and the object are treated in the same way.

## 5. CONCLUSIONS

I cannot, unfortunately, elaborate on this clinical case. It illustrates the difficulty in maintaining distance and establishing a constructive connection with this type of patient. Luckily, certain borderlines are more open to introjection and respond to analysis. Sometimes the setting must be modified.

In conclusion, I will say that the mechanisms of massive projective identification are at work. The analyst, like any other object, becomes the container for essential elements of the patient which he or she evacuates. The working-through process where representations, memories and renewals - through the integration of affect - in cases with a favourable prognosis - allow the ego of the patient to be reinforced and more effective boundaries to be established.

Thought also serves as a link to the lost object once and then a thousand times over, because of the anal treatment to which it has been subjected.

Borderline thought disorders are the result, in my opinion, of attacks on internal objects, identified as objects in transference, which result in a mental void, feelings of emptiness, of nothingness.

The anal structure of these patients varies greatly. They may be very rigid, establishing boundaries through obsessional defences. Sometimes they become inconsistent, bordering on confusion. When boundaries are broken down, acting out, chaos or internal disorganisation makes its appearance. In successful cases, they are replaced by more effective organisation with more adequate defences, after analysis.

# Narcissism and Society

Juan Manzano
*President, Swiss Psychoanalytical Society*

The links between intra-psychic, social and cultural issues are undeniable. Freud's entire work reflects his interest in these issues, and other analysts have followed in his footsteps. When the behaviour of a social group is clearly characterised by its alienation, *i.e.* by a breakdown in its relations with reality, together with the potential or overt destructiveness of its acts, it is my belief that psychoanalysts can contribute by proposing models that may help us to understand and change the group. I am thinking of phenomena such as attitudes to nuclear weapons, ecological disasters, nationalism, *etc.*

I intend to present for discussion a model of narcissism that can be applied to social phenomena. It is part of a broader clinical study I have undertaken with F. Palacio (2001).

## 1. MULTI-AXIAL MODEL OF NARCISSISM

In this theoretical model, each axis represents one of the relatively autonomous concepts encompassed by the notion of narcissism. But since it is also a developmental model, the same axes show the evolution of each of these aspects from their most archaic or infantile form to the most mature. In addition, the model is a clinical one, whose aim is to provide us with a profile of psychic functioning from the point of view of narcissism.

### 1.1 Instinctual Axis

It is generally accepted that the narcissistic libido predominates in early childhood and that the object-libido gradually takes over, resulting in what Grumberger (1971) has called a «synthesis solution» between the narcissistic libido and the object-libido, corresponding to each evolution of the personality.

The predominance of the narcissistic libido over the object-libido manifests itself, in particular, by conscious and unconscious fantasies, but also by relational behaviour. These fantasies and behaviour represent the various ways in which the narcissistic libido seeks satisfaction: admiration, megalomania, feeling of unicity, search for uniformity, and negation of the generation gap.

Without going into the second theory of instinct here, the existence of fantasies and aggressive behaviour and their progression during the development of narcissism from a moment when the object is ignored (negation, denial) to fantasies and behaviour of direct object aggression, is fairly widely accepted.

## 1.2 Object-relationship and Self-axis

Whether or not we accept the fact that there is a phase without an object (primary narcissism), there is a clinical consensus around the fact that there is always an early idealisation of the object and, consequently, a relationship with this ideal object. This early, narcissistic type of relationship is expressed by fusional fantasies with the ideal object (or fantasy of projective identification) and by its correlate of a total, then partial lack of differentiation with this ideal object. As development progresses and as it becomes impossible to deny the separation and existence of the object in external reality, several vicissitudes of the narcissistic relationship appear, together with various narcissistic fantasies, including envy of the idealised object.

This narcissistic object relationship predominates early on and would seem to develop at the same time as the anaclitic object relationship cathected with object-libido. Here too, there is usually a progression towards a «synthesis solution» of the narcissistic and object relationships, where the object relationship predominates.

## 1.3 Axis Relating to the Mechanisms Regulating Self-esteem

It is possible to distinguish a clear developmental trend going from immature (infantile) mechanisms of regulation to more evolved ones (adults). The former are characterised mainly by their dependence on the attitude of the cathected object, the latter by the relationship of the ego with, on the one hand, the part of it that has been differentiated into an ideal ego (or ego-ideal) left over from narcissism and, on the other hand, with a realistic perception of its own efficiency to adapt and obtain satisfaction.

## 1.4 Cognitive Axis

From a developmental point of view, the most important point is the differentiation of one's representation of the self and of the object, and the consequences the vicissitudes of this differentiation have on the whole of the thought process.

## 1.5 Structure of Personality Axis

All authors seem to agree on the basic characteristics of pathological narcissistic personalities, both from a clinical and a relational point of view. They also agree on the types of transference and processes that characterise patients of this type in analysis or in psychotherapy.

Here too we can follow a developmental axis. As we have already stated, there is thought to be a narcissistic withdrawal of the libido, predominating in the first stages of childhood. This withdrawal has a mainly defensive purpose against paranoid anxieties in particular, and is thus linked to a structure similar to the one described by Kernberg (1975) in adult pathology: splitting of the ego, with a «narcissistic» part (identified with the ideal object) and an «inferior», «negative» or «aggressive» part, projected into the external object and denied. Later, these primitive defences evolve towards a lessening of the splitting, leading to a greater integration of the ego. At this stage, the narcissistic withdrawal acts as a defence against the depressive anxieties of separation and loss of the object.

# 2. AN EXAMPLE OF APPLICATION OF THE MODEL TO SOCIAL PHENOMENA: NATIONALISM

The multi-axial model of narcissism I have just outlined can also be applied to social phenomena such as nationalism and the various forms it takes: racist, religious, linguistic, *etc*. It is obvious that other factors such as socio-economic factors, historical factors or group factors are involved in the emergence of nationalist movements. The interests of the outsiders and the presence of leaders pursuing their own goals usually have also to be taken into consideration. Nevertheless, independently of the particular place, time and circumstances, we find *common reaction patterns* in nationalist group members. These common patterns can be understood in terms of narcissism.

It is as if people who are subjected to these group conditions regress, more or less deeply, towards archaic, narcissistic structures.

I now propose to give a brief analysis of these common reaction patterns using our multi-axial model.

## 2.1 Instinctual Axis

We observe the presence of more or less conscious «megalomaniac» fantasies and of behaviour tending to satisfy these fantasies. Even when not stated explicitly or even consciously, the person always has to feel superior, better, if not unique. We also find fantasies of uniformity, of homogenisation: the group members must be equal, identical, thus denying or minimising any differences or possible conflicts within the group.
The fantasies and the aggressive, destructive behaviour are aimed at «the others», the outsiders («strange», «inferior», «lacking a soul»). These outsiders must be carefully identified, often on the basis of «small», existing «differences» (religion, language, colour of skin, *etc.*) or even totally fabricated ones. In our opinion, violent behaviour is rooted in the need to turn into a reality the obvious projection into the other person of everything that is intrinsically different from the idealised criteria of the group. In addition to being «inferior», the outsider is «instinctual» and, therefore, menacing and aggressive. He/she thus becomes anti-narcissistic and must be destroyed, because of their very existence.

## 2.2 Object Relationship Axis

The members of these groups thus tend to form narcissistic libidinal relationships: undifferentiated within the group, *they become a confused ideal* within this ideal group (pure, spotless, in perfect harmony). The relationship with «the others» is aggressive.

## 2.3 Axis Relating to the Mechanism Regulating Self-esteem

Self-esteem is regulated by the infantile mechanism of dependence on the attitudes of the group. The members self-assert themselves reciprocally.

## 2.4 Cognitive Axis

This functioning leads inevitably to thought disorders, which can be observed in the elaboration of ideological, historical or social structures that have little or no contact with reality. Reality is distorted in order to give satisfaction to narcissistic fantasies. The relation with reality is replaced by «reciprocal self-confirmations» between the members of the group, and by the very real perception of the consequences of their destructive acts on others.

## 2.5 Personality Structure Axis

It seems quite clear that the members of nationalist groups tend to regress to the «paranoid, narcissistic structures» described above. These are characterised by: a splitting of the ego into an idealised part identified with all the other members of the group, and an «inferior», «negative», «aggressive» part projected onto the others, who insofar as they cannot simply be denied, becoming menacing and persecutory. The mechanism leading to violence described above is thus sparked off and becomes inevitable.

# 3. CONCLUSION

I think that this model, which can be expressed in simple language, understandable to the layman, could serve as a bridge for dialogue and collaboration with the social sciences.

**References**

Grunberger, B., 1971, *Le Narcissisme*, Paris, Payot

Kernberg, O., 1975, *Borderline Conditions and Pathological Narcissism*. N.Y. Jason Aronson

Manzano, J. Palacio, E. *Narcissisme paranoïde et narcissisme dépressif. Un modèle multiaxial du narcissisme* (forthcoming publication)

# Psychoanalysis and Health

Robert Michels
*American Psychoanalytical Society*

There are a number of issues at the interface of psychoanalysis and health, ranging from the very origin of psychoanalysis to current threats to its future. I will discuss them under five headings: (1) History, (2) Theory, (3) Clinical, (4) Social, and (5) Professional.

## 1. HISTORY

Psychoanalysis started in the relationship between a physician and his patients seeking treatment for problems of health. The intimacy of the doctor-patient relationship, the trust that patients place in their physicians, and the scope of a physician's interest in his patient's experiences provided the essential context for Freud's discoveries and for the birth of psychoanalysis.

As we know, Freud was later concerned lest the method he had developed might be seen as merely one more method of treatment in psychiatry. He was adamant that psychoanalytic institutes should be independent of medical schools (or even universities) and that psychoanalysts did not have to be psychiatrists, or even physicians. Of course the question of health is behind all of these issues—if psychoanalysis is a treatment designed to make sick people healthy, at least at first glance it would seem to belong in a medical school and to be a treatment administered by psychiatrists.

This health orientation to psychoanalysis was, in spite of Freud, most popular for many years in the United States, where psychoanalysis flourished in medicine and psychiatry, was seen as a treatment for mental disorders, and was distinctly unfriendly to non-medical would-be psychoanalysts. In recent years this health orientation has diminished and American psychoanalysis has become less health oriented, and thus more like psychoanalysis in the rest of the world. However this was significantly in response to external challenges and threats; the underlying questions of the appropriate relation of psychoanalysis to health have not been resolved, but rather deferred.

## 2. THEORY

Freud saw psychoanalysis as uncovering the causes of neurotic phenomena and, in so doing, modifying them. Sandor Rado, Heinz Hartmann and others recognised that this was fundamentally a biologic conceptualisation, that the adaptation of the organism and its fitting into the environment was a fundamental framework for psychoanalysis, and that this inevitably raised questions of health. Psychoanalysts were interested in adaptation, psychoanalytic treatment could enhance adaptation, and optimal adaptation was synonymous with health.

In recent years many psychoanalysts have questioned Freud's understanding of what psychoanalysis is. They have challenged both his biology and his epistemology, and have suggested that psychoanalysis is a method for exploring meanings rather than discovering causes—a hermeneutic discipline rather than a scientific one. In this view psychoanalysis is concerned with fantasies and symbols, with the personal meanings with which individuals envelop the facts of their lives rather than with these facts themselves. It is a method of exegesis and translation, not of treatment or cure. As such it would be neutral to health.

## 3. CLINICAL

Today most psychoanalysts are more interested in clinical than historical or theoretical issues—what psychoanalysts do with patients and how their ideas affect what they do, rather than philosophic or definitional concerns. Considerations of health are important at several points in the course of clinical work.

First, for some, health or sickness has to do with the indications for psychoanalysis. Patients (a health-oriented term) become analysands because analysis is prescribed (another health-oriented term) for their problems. In this view, analysis is a medical or psychiatric treatment, parallel to other treatments, for ill health.

However there is evidence that most analysts don't simply think this way, for they are more likely to discuss analysability—the patient's capacity to participate in the analysis—than whether or not the patient has a disease that is best treated by analysis. Medical doctors think differently. They spend far more time discussing the best treatment for a given problem than whether the patient is suitable for the treatment. It is rare to hear of an analyst turning away an unanalysed yet analysable person who is interested in analysis simply because the person doesn't have an appropriate problem that should be treated by analysis. However if, as this suggests, analysis is for everyone who can participate in it, then it is unlike any other treatments related to health, except perhaps preventive measures like immunisation or vitamins.

Nevertheless, analysts do think about health at times other than when evaluating potential analysands. Patients may develop health problems—either mental or somatic—in the course of analysis. The analysts then must evaluate whether this is something to be understood in terms of meanings, transference, communication and thus analysed, or as a possibly important but independent event, or as a toxic side effect of the analysis itself—one that might call for a clinical reassessment, interruption, change in technique, initiation of an additional «co» therapy, or even termination, to prevent further negative impact.

Health will also be a consideration for many analysts when contemplating termination. Is the patient «better», are symptoms diminished, is adaptation enhanced? Has the «treatment» led to a «cure»?

Finally, if health values are prominent in the analyst's mind when the termination is being considered, they must be in the background the rest of the time. Analysts who believe that they are trying to improve their patients' health will hear their patients' material through a health-related filter. In the inevitable decisions of the clinical process, they will select issues and themes that seem linked to the patient's pathology. Indeed some define psychoanalytic psychotherapy as employing many of the methods of psychoanalysis, but always with the specific intention of improving the patient's health. If one wants to treat sick people, one actively searches for the signs and symptoms of disease. If the healer and the interpreter are faced with the same individual, one creates a patient, the other an analysand, each in concordance with his pre-existing organising framework.

## 4. SOCIAL

Society is concerned about the qualifications and the ethics of those charged with caring for the sick. This leads to various forms of credentialing and licensure, along with barriers that prevent practice by those who are not part of a profession or are viewed as unqualified. There is no such concern about practitioners who suggest alternate meanings for personal experience, but do not present themselves as treating diseases—religious figures, fortune tellers, astrologers, palm readers and the like. The psychoanalytic profession has been ambivalent on this issue, wanting some of the privileges that accompany the responsibility of caring for the sick, but being unwilling to accept some of the social regulations and constraints that are corollaries.

Perhaps the most critical social privilege today stems from the belief in many communities that the costs of treatment for the sick should be subsidised by public resources. Practically speaking, this has immense impact on the availability of psychoanalysis to the public, and on the rewards of a psychoanalytic career. In contrast, no one has suggested that public support is appropriate for a process of personal discovery that is not employed to treat those who are sick. The relation of psychoanalysis to health is closely tied to the relation of psychoanalysis to public support.

## 5. PROFESSIONAL

Professions are organised groups of individuals who have special knowledge and skills that are useful to society and that are accorded privileges and autonomy in their area of expertise. Health care disciplines such as medicine and nursing are classical professions. Professionals are considered responsible not only for their personal services but also for assuring the public of the quality of services provided by colleagues, for educating future professionals, for advancing the field by acquiring new knowledge, and for advising the public in their area of competence.

Here again psychoanalysis has been ambivalent. Analysts have been slow to accept collective responsibility for the quality of care offered by others who call themselves analysts, and unlike the health professions, have even failed to develop clear boundaries delineating who is and who is not an analyst. Intensely interested in education, they have been less attentive to research or the acquisition of new knowledge. Some believe that psychoanalysis is on the verge of becoming a true profession, others that it should be a specialisation of several existing professions (medicine, clinical psychology, social work, *etc.*) and still others that the restrictions, bureaucratisation and public control involved in a profession threaten more than they offer, and that something essential to psychoanalysis is best preserved if it remains unique.

Two concrete issues that have long concerned psychoanalysis can be traced to its relation to health and the health professions. Both have recurred throughout its history. One is the appropriate relationship between psychoanalytic institutes and universities. Most professional schools are linked to universities, and the growth of knowledge that leads to progress in the professions is greatly enhanced by those linkages. Psychoanalytic institutes are different—they are largely independent. The other issue is the appropriate prerequisites for psychoanalytic training. The early discussion about lay analysis took place in a world of physicians and laymen. That world has changed, so that we now have psychiatrists, social workers, clinical nurses, counsellors and others, all considering themselves health professionals, but neither laymen nor physicians. We also have humanists, scholars, academics, teachers and others with intense interest in psychoanalysis, often considerable knowledge regarding its concepts and theories, but no experience in issues of health and no professional socialisation. Should they be trained as psychoanalysts? Do they require remedial education in health? Can psychoanalytic training alone provide professional socialisation equivalent to that of the health professions? If not, is such socialisation necessary? Should limitations be placed on their appropriate scope of practice? These questions have not been answered, and at times it seems as though the profession has avoided them in order to avoid internal conflict.

## 6. FUTURE

I can only offer a personal view of the relationship between psychoanalysis and health today, and the direction that it might take in the future. The psychoanalytic method has evolved and developed partly as a treatment for psychiatric disorders and partly as a method of exploration in situations with little relationship to health, examining both persons and their creations with little concern for pathology. It has been effective and productive in each of these domains, and will continue to be so, with the psychoanalytic process serving both as a treatment and as a means for personal growth and enhancement. What we learn in each arena enhances our work in the other. However regardless of the domain, concern with health and with the body is central to the human condition, and knowledge of these subjects is essential for anyone intending to practice psychoanalysis. Those who would use it as a treatment for health problems must have more. If they are to prescribe analysis for patients they must be educated in alternative treatments, and in the reasons for selecting one or the other. If they are to use psychoanalysis in order to treat patients for problems of health, they should be members of a recognised profession, and be thoroughly socialised as health professionals. At present, psychoanalytic training itself does not provide this socialisation. It may develop it in the future, or it may continue to rely on the prior socialisation of other health professions.

There may be analysts, and excellent ones, who do not fulfil these qualifications. I believe either that their practice should be limited to the non-health based domain of analysis or that they must be monitored and regulated very carefully. Without this, the public will not trust psychoanalysis as a profession and will not provide public support for the psychoanalytic treatment of patients.

Finally, the reasons for separating psychoanalysis from the university have long ceased to be relevant, and the continued cost of that separation has been particularly great to the health-related functions of analysis. It is vital that we learn which patients are helped more by psychoanalysis than by other treatments, and which are not, and how to make analysis more helpful. This kind of inquiry is not really psychoanalytic science, it is rather the scientific study of the effects of psychoanalysis. It requires work by psychoanalysts, but it also requires collaboration by experts in other disciplines, experts that are readily available in universities and rarely outside of them.

## 7. CONCLUSIONS

My own view is that psychoanalysis is based on a central paradox—it is a medically derived treatment that requires for its success the suspension of external therapeutic goals. Even when it has been prescribed as a treatment for a problem of health, it is best conducted as an inquiry that proceeds without concern for health or pathology in order to focus on the search for meaning. Psychoanalysts at their best exercise health expertise in deciding whom to analyse, and perhaps when to stop, and psychoanalytic expertise in being able to keep these issues at bay while conducting the analysis. If questions of health do emerge in the clinical material they should be regarded first and foremost as countertransference signals.

# From Medicine to Psychoanalysis and Psychosomatics

*Psyche and Soma*

Marilia Aisenstein
*Paris Psychoanalytical Society*

Various philosophical and theological responses have been proposed to get beyond the idea that thought is necessarily mortal, since it is tied to the body. Hence the notion of an immortal soul, the seat of thought, not reducible to the uncertainties of the soma. Here I offer some semantic considerations: "soma", the Greek word for body, took on its present sense of a living organism only during the Fifth and Fourth centuries B.C. with Hippocrates. Before the *Corpus Hypocratum,* the term soma referred to an inanimate body or corpse. "Psyche" originally signified breath and, by extension, the breath of life and then soul. It is worth recalling that these semantic shifts occurred at a time when Hippocrates was founding medicine as a scientific discipline based on objective observation and the study of symptoms (semiology).

Depending on whether or not psyche-soma is seen as singular or dual, one may construct different systems explaining man and the world, life and death. To take a strictly Freudian stance, the emergence of thought was initiated by the sight of a corpse that was both loved and hated, provoking the double thought: "may it go away" and "I want to keep it as it is". Traces of this initial conflict allow thought to partake of immortality, opening the way to speculation on death and life, life which endures longer than a generation.

The discoveries of psychoanalysis offer, in my view, a perfectly cogent and unique solution to the famous mind/body problem, the dualism psyche/soma. In transferring the duality psyche-soma, onto the duality of drives, psychoanalysis places the origin of the thought process in the initial conflict. The very definition of drives - a psychical processing of a sexual somatic excitation - confirms, in the two theories of drives, a psychophysical parallel to which Freud had drawn attention as early as 1891.

Human beings are "psychosomatic": if every thought is, as Tertullian (c150 A.D. to c220 A.D) wrote, an "act of the flesh", all pain and all pleasure are also psychical acts. The Freudian description of the hallucination of pleasure as an expectation and distance necessary for desire is a sign of this. The field of what one might today call psychosomatic practice (the psychoanalytic approach to patients afflicted with somatic disorders) was not discussed by Freud although he was to lay its foundations.

In *Beyond the Pleasure Principle* (1920; English edition Norton, N.Y. 1961), an essay which inaugurated the second functional dualism, thereby founding the second topography, Freud, after distinguishing between "pure" and organic-lesional traumas, noted that the existence of a circumscribed lesion seemed to protect the subject from the emergence of a traumatic neurosis. Here Freud discusses the drastic effect of a painful somatic illness on the distribution and modalities of the libido.

The violence of the mechanical trauma liberates a quantum of excitation which is all the more disorganising in that there has been no preparation for it by anxiety. However, the occurrence of a physical lesion may allow an incorporation of the excess excitation through a "narcissistic hypercathexis" of the affected organ. On the basis of these remarks, Freud notes that pathognomonic mental symptoms such as melancholia or even chronic dementia praecox may temporarily disappear during an intercurrent organic disorder.

The above discussion provides a starting point for our present psychosomatic approach.

## 1. A LOGICAL DEVELOPMENT OF PSYCHO-ANALYSIS: THE PARIS PSYCHOSOMATIC SCHOOL

While the perception of health in terms of a psycho-somatic balance has its origins in Hippocratic medicine, the current of thought underlying the Paris Psychosomatic School stems from the discovery of the psychoanalytic method. It is not the place here to go into the history of successive psychosomatic theories, but I would like to stress that our form of psychosomatics is fundamentally a logical outcome of psychoanalysis; I would even claim that in some ways it is its culmination.

In answer to the psyche-soma enigma, Freud proposed a remarkable reply which I would summarise as follows: "The confrontation is not between the body and its desires on one side and psyche and its wishes on the other; rather, contradictory forces may come into conflict at a single somatic site."

In his 1910 essay *A Psycho-analytic View of a Psychogenic Disturbance of Vision* (S.E. vol. 11), Freud raised the idea of an organ forced simultaneously to serve two masters; it is this conflict that gives meaning to an organic symptom. It is worth noting that this text has a special status: since the research model of the period was one of neurosis, Freud wrote little about psychogenesis. Hysterical conversion makes the body into a language, the symptoms telling an unconscious story, and all mental activity finds its sources in the erotic libido. The question of psychogenesis versus organo-genesis is thus not a truly psychoanalytic one.

Moreover, the strictly etiological approach would, I feel, always be reductionist. If, faced with the clinical picture of hysteria, Freud chose to disregard the taboo surrounding the psychical component of certain disorders, he did so in a way that illustrates the vital importance of the sexual - hence the body - in the constitution of the psyche.

Dreams, the royal road to analytic science, can only be understood with reference to the sleep of a particular individual. Dreams integrate exogenous and endogenous somatic stimulations in the working through of a psychical process aimed primarily at the success of a physiological function, namely the pursuit of sleep. The interest of psychoanalysis in dreams shows the importance of the somatic dimension in all psychic work. Although psychoanalysis began in opposition to the medical and neurological thought of the 19th century, it is nonetheless intrinsically bound up with physiology. The psychoanalytic treatment of patients suffering from somatic disorders is hence a return to the very sources of the psychoanalytic quest.

Here I will say just a few words about the theoretical model elaborated by the Paris Psychosomatic School (Pierre Marty, Michel de M'Uzan, Michel Fain, Christian David)(1) beginning in the 1950s.

After establishing the psychosomatic unity of the human being and the principle of economy, this approach allows psychical and somatic phenomena to be understood as a sum of dynamic interactions which are the object of movements of organisation and disorganisation. Although it may have no symbolic meaning, somatic disorder may be part of a general economy in which the psyche is both witness and controller.

In this model, instinctual drives have their source in bodily excitations. Their role is to deal with the tensions thus created. If the sum of excitations continues to be excessive, the functional systems become disorganised, the mental apparatus overloaded, leaving the way open to somatisation. The notions of disorganisation, fixation and regression, are hence central to this extremely coherent and complex conception which is difficult to summarise in a few words.

I will start by pointing out that Pierre Marty and his colleagues from various disciplines - neurosurgery, gastroenterology, internal medicine and psychoanalysis - had been struck by the absence of any mental symptomatology in the course of a somatic disease. This observation ties in with a remark by Freud who in 1920 referred to a "psychical cure" during an intercurrent psychical illness. The "distribution of libido must be involved" he notes (S.E. vol. 18, page 23). From this observation, one may deduce the protective role that mental defence systems, be they neurotic, psychotic or perverse, may play. Their insufficiency or absence opens the way to a somatic excitation that cannot be worked through by the psyche.

In organised psychoses as well as in well-established neurotic structures such as we all have, illness upsets the habitual system as a result of the withdrawal of the libido and its necessary transformation into a narcissistic libido.

On the other hand, there is a whole range of poorly structured psychical organisations caused by deficiencies or early trauma. In such cases, character traits or attachment to narcissistic values replace strictly mental defences. Recourse to a somatic solution is frequent; this short circuits any psychical working through such as acting out by borderline patients.

This phenomenon is what has been described as "alexithymia" (by Sifnéos and Namias in the U.S.) and as "*pensée opératoire*", "mechanical thought" or "mechanical functioning" (by P.Marty and M. de M'Uzan in France).

In different contexts, the two terms refer to the same clinical entity *i.e.* an absence of mental symptoms, a lack of affect, anxiety, and thought which is objective rather than metaphorical, as if cut off from a system of representations.

We are talking here of a new field which gives the psychoanalyst greater scope for action but at the same time imposes the use of different technical parameters.

Following Winnicot, I would say in regard to the technical implications that: "*the practice of psychoanalysis also includes psychotherapy*" as well as the modifications necessary for patients' psychical organisation.

The present extension of the psychoanalytical method to "non-neurotic", borderline and psychotic patients as well as to those who are physically ill, shows that the standard treatment model is often inapplicable as such in our daily practice. Changes in setting and in interpretive techniques do not imply any move away from rigorous psychoanalytical practice aimed at eliciting transference. I would add in passing that handling these difficult therapies requires a long experience of classical psychoanalysis. If one is to be flexible *vis-a-vis* a particular model, one must first have assimilated it completely.

There are many technical considerations that need to be taken into account when treating such cases in a psychoanalytic framework. Face-to-face sessions are frequently indicated inasmuch as they facilitate adaptation to the affective state of the patients. It must be remembered that patients do not always come on their own initiative; they are often sent by specialists who "prescribe" a psychoanalytic psychotherapy. They have to be met on their own ground. Above all, they need to be given support in the early stages by the analyst who must constantly be aware of possible qualitative alterations in mental functioning.

The inefficacy of secondary narcissism and patients' lack of commitment to treatment make the task of interpretation difficult. The use of associative techniques may, on the other hand, serve to access various topics and engage in a "conversation".

I use the term "conversation" advisedly, as I believe that in every psychoanalytic psychotherapy of this type, there is an approach that I would call the "art of conversation". To interest patients in the thought process, one must think with them and involve them in the process. I would even go so far as to talk of a kind of "seduction" that tries to make the patient realise that nobody has nothing to say, no life is without its story and no story without its words, its richness and its sorrows. Topics that are apparently nonconflictual like literature, cinema, and current affairs, although providing only an indirect approach, do allow one to locate regressive movements, tolerance of excitation, and disorganising effects. Recourse to what I would call "psychodramatic interpretations" (of the type "If I were you....") both respects the narcissism of the patient and opens up possibilities of identification. Everything should be done to support and stimulate pre-conscious work and thereby help patients to discover and share in the pleasure of mental functioning.

Here I will present a brief example.

## 2. CLINICAL MATERIAL

Claire was a high-ranking research chemist working in the French civil service. Slim and willowy, with pleasant features and blond curls, this 32-year old, might have been most attractive were it not for a touch of blandness. Dressed plainly, she was not exactly dull but lacked sparkle. There was something blurred and misty about her; she reminded me of an early Odilon Redon. She had been sent to me by her then cardiologist who, like many of his predecessors, seemed to have been discouraged by his lack of success in controlling Claire's labile hypertension. When she came to me, poised but somewhat shy, I realised that this patient must have managed to show a particularly unappealing side of herself to have produced such untoward reactions on the part of her doctors.

These reactions could not have been explained simply by the failure of the treatment. In what she recounted to me, there was no pathological truculence. She spoke without any manifestation of sadness or humour. There was a lot she didn't understand, and I felt a deep sense of hurt. She had come to psychotherapy, not out of any great belief in it but because she wanted to embark on a third pregnancy, and this had been advised against on medical grounds. She felt that her life was empty. Professionally she was doing well, but she got no sense of pride from her career. She had taken up pharmacy on the advice of her parents and continued on with an *agrégation* in chemistry. She pursued her studies without difficulty but without passion.

Claire recounted an exemplary existence. The only daughter of a couple of prominent citizens (who had wanted a child), she had gone to school in a religious establishment. Her father was a university lecturer in German while her mother had looked after her daughter's education. There were few outings and no friends in her provincial childhood. Her parents made her read, play the piano and visit museums. Her holidays and leisure time were spent in cultural pursuits, but these seemed to have little impact on Claire who was no great reader and showed no interest in the arts.

Claire's husband was also a scientist, from one of France's most prestigious schools. They married young and soon had two sons who were doing well. Her mother and father had died seven and five years ago respectively.

Claire's hypertension was first detected, thanks to a school medical when she was 13. Claire recalled little of this dull and uneventful time; the only thing she remembers worrying about were pains and swelling in her breasts. Her mother had taken her to the family doctor, a retired colonel, who had been astonished to have to explain to them that Claire was starting puberty. Claire recounted this without any amusement or any criticism of her mother, but what struck her was the baffled expression of the doctor. Later I was to observe the frequency of her astonishment at the expressions she provoked in others, which she could not decode but to which she reacted with anxiety. In my view, she had an alarming inability to identify with others, and this helped me to better understand her relational difficulties. Claire's socio-professional level and the quality of her vocabulary were in such marked contrast to the deficiencies in her pre-conscious system that she was often the object of projective mechanisms. Her inability to perceive ambiguities in a particular word or situation made it impossible for her to understand the most obvious jokes. This was seen by others as rigidity.

This "alexithymia", to use the term coined by Sifnéos, both in regard to oneself and to others, goes hand-in-hand with a permanent state of alarm and hurt which, though not expressed, I can often sense. The absence of any space for identification play, together with an incomplete secondary narcissism and thus the absence of self-esteem, along with the absence of any system of mental defence leads to major technical difficulties in effecting a cure. A face-to-face analysis, which obliges the patient to confront otherness in the person of the analyst, is essential here in promoting the work of "reanimation" and the modulation of emotional states by means of suggested scenarios or explanations. Rather than being imposed on patients in a direct, interpretive form, these may simply be proposed and, depending on the emotions provoked, be modified as necessary. A face-to-face analysis with pre-conscious working through by the therapist provides the necessary support but may confront patients with what they feel to be their incompleteness. A sentence of the type: "Once again I hadn't understood" may be corrected by the analyst with an identificatory proposition (psychodramatic technique) of the type: "Don't worry if you find it difficult to follow my reasoning. Can you imagine how lost I would be trying to understand your chemical equations?"

These modalities or technical specifics are designed to give constant support to damaged or frozen psychical work; at the same time they encourage the development of psychic material in the course of analysis. In this way, a story is woven together that will eventually become transference. At the rate of one session per week and as the years went by, the story of Claire's psychotherapy was constructed between the two of us. The maturing of the relationship allowed occasional interpretations in the transference: when she was telling me about a film, I suggested to her that "today it is you who are saying these words for me".

Three years passed. There was a slight improvement in her symptoms: hypertension surges had become less frequent, and Claire had come to enjoy the sessions and was trying to connect her thoughts, present and past.

One day, when she was telling me about her childhood, I was troubled by the poverty of the images she was evoking in me; these were frozen, and their details were curiously repetitive. I decided to tell her my feelings and said: "I have the impression you are thumbing through an old photo album." Claire was suddenly taken aback and told me that as a child she had wondered why there were no photos at home. Shortly afterwards, other forgotten questions came back to her: her mother said that she was from eastern France, but had never said from which town. At the oral examination of the *baccalauréat*, she had been called by a double name, her own, with some other she was not familiar with. I mentioned that this name had a Jewish ring, and I remembered that Claire had been born during the war.

I will summarise below the next four years devoted to the search for her identity and the discovery of her Jewishness. In the course of a long trip to meet a relative about whom she knew only that he existed, she learnt that her real father, who had died in the camps, was the brother of her supposed father. Under Mosaic law, the latter had married her mother and recognised the child as his own. Their French name was chosen before the family, under the pressure of events, converted. Claire became quite excited at this discovery of a past which had been hidden from her and read as much as she could to fill in the gaps. Analysis became more attractive; more associations were made and the process became more classical. Claire decided to embark on a third pregnancy and a daughter was born whom she called Esther. Married life, however, deteriorated. Her husband became a stranger with whom she had little in common.

Some months later, we began the third phase of this psychotherapy which was to last in all 11 years. After a time of elation, Claire became seriously depressed. Working through her triple mourning and its inherent uncertainties represented the positive aspect of this depression which nonetheless persisted to a point where I became sufficiently alarmed to send her to a psychiatrist colleague. He prescribed a low dose of anti-depressants, and Claire was so satisfied that she decided to continue with this treatment. At the same time, she announced that her blood pressure had become perfectly normal without medication. I was wondering about the link between the two phenomena when her cardiologist called me to tell of his puzzlement at the remission of her symptoms upon taking anti-depressants. I questioned Claire on her psychical and bodily experience in regard to medication. It was then, and with much reticence, that she admitted that she had always felt profoundly ill at ease when not in a hyper-tense state. The feeling of internal flabbiness and lethargy terrified her. Passivity in general horrified her. In fact, she had taken her beta blockers only in tiny doses which she herself had divided up.

During her depression and, even though her blood pressure had come down, the anti-depressants gave her a vague sense of excitement - she called it "tonus" - which she liked. This confession which came during our tenth year of psychoanalysis, was to be the starting point of our final phase. The examination of her intolerance to all forms of passive satisfaction threw fresh and final light on her specific Oedipal organisation.

I have recounted here a long adventure which included sudden passionate outpourings but also moments of despair; I wonder if the latter would have been tolerable without constant recourse to a theory which lends support to the technical creativity of the analyst.

## 3. A PERSONAL THEORETICAL CONSIDERATION

I now invite you to follow me in seeing psychoanalysis as a fresh and original response to the old question of psyche/soma, the other face of the primal question: how can intelligence (or the soul) be immortal and survive a body that is by definition mortal.

I would say that Freud's true subversion is his conception of the human condition that anchors thought in a sexual finitude, all the more finite in that it is sexualised *i.e.* cut or divided (*c.f.* the Latin *secare* - to divide).

Thought is defined here not as language or discourse in the philosophical sense, but as a container of metaphorical and visual space. Thought is incarnate, rooted in the body.

Psychoanalysis involves the "working out of thought"; it modifies every thought about thought. In my view, the true revolution at the heart of psychoanalysis dates from 1920 with *Beyond the Pleasure Principle*.

The first instinctual opposition already places the conflict at the heart of the psyche, shifting it away from the polarity body/mind. This theory of drives gets round the question of destruction and death by separating sexuality and self-preservation into antagonistic forces. The conceptual and philosophical impasse of this debate, like Freud's ethical hesitations after the

Great War and the introduction of the notion of narcissism, led him to reformulate his earlier meta-psychology which, in any case, was inadequate to account for clinical failures.

Faced with, on the one hand, an epistemological difficulty and, on the other, with the difficulties he experienced in dealing with repetition-compulsion and negative therapeutic reaction and in analysing psychoses and trauma, Freud was obliged to call into question his conception of drives in favour of narcissism and a destructive drive whose force he had perhaps failed to appreciate. The second theory of drives was now inevitable. This second conflict of drives between the libido, which brings together sexuality and self-preservation, and the death drive is for me of particular interest in that it represents a new formulation of the fundamentals.

The debate is no longer about whether sexuality is on the side of life or death but about placing this opposition within the very processes of thought. In my view it is crucial to re-centre the question of death and replace it at the centre of thought, since the primary opposition is that of the human condition - by definition mortal - unique in its capacity to think what is eternal. The act of thinking would thus carry in itself the denial of mortality and finitude. The death drive, as I see it, is not only defusion, in opposition to Eros, as defined in the *Outline* of 1939 (published in 1940), but that which, from within the psyche, constantly threatens all work of thinking. This "death" drive has nothing to do with inevitable organic death but is to be envisaged rather as a principle of psychical death which, in the form of a motion, or even of a disincarnating force, attacks and kills thought at the very heart of the thought process.

Like the worm in the fruit, or even the pearl in the oyster, a metaphor which Freud employed to illustrate that in every defence psychoneurosis lies the germ of the actual neurosis, the psyche carries within itself its own tendency to destroy the work of thought. If we are to think of the depressive position and the working through of mourning as carriers of psychical elaboration, we are led to wonder if there is not, within every depressive movement, a potential risk of attack against the psyche. The "*pensée opératoire*" (mechanical thought or functioning) described by the adherents of the Paris School of Psychosomatics would be an extreme and exemplary case of this form of destruction, in other words a system of anti-dream discourse.

## 4. CONCLUSIONS

I conclude this discussion by stressing once again that behind the ordinariness of simple phenomena may lie quite complex causes and that our theories are not to be taken as truths but rather as constructions that help us to think and assist our patients. I would add that the practice of psychoanalysis and, *a fortiori*, psychoanalytic psychosomatics should teach us to be modest because what we know is minimal compared with the vastness of the questions that have yet to be answered.

# Psychoanalysis and Primary Health Care

*Our Participation as Psychoanalysts in a Long-overdue Change in the Health Services*

Jorge L. Tizón
*Spanish Psychoanalytical Society*

## 1. PRIMARY HEALTH CARE

From a health care point of view, the second half of the 20th century, and especially the 1960s and 1970s, brought with it a significant rise in the number of visible problems in modern Western medicine and in its exportation to the countries of the 'Second' and 'Third Worlds'. Certain counter-cultural criticisms have also underlined some of the more difficult to solve shortcomings of the dominant health-care system. These criticisms include those of the French May of 1968 movement, those of Ivan Illich (1975), those of traditional medicines in many countries, those of revolutionary health organisations, such as the Spanish (1931-1939), the Chinese, the Cuban, and so on.

At the same time, also during the same period, a creative parallel and afterwards convergent movement was developed *from general practice*, from British *general practitioners* and American *general physicians*, and by some *paediatricians of social or psychosocial orientation*. This movement coincided with other types of - very different - criticisms and contributions, coming in this case from economists, health service administrators, politicians and more- or less-alternative leaders. From one side or the other they criticised the unstoppable costs of the system, its bureaucratisation, its lack of equality and solidarity, its inefficacy, inefficiency, lack of safety, inaccessibility, its strengthening of the heteronomy of patients, rather than their autonomy (a basic component of health) and so on. In 'underdeveloped' countries, budget insufficiencies of the health systems themselves were criticised as well as their orientation and their ways of working, which involved the crushing of native cultures and medicines. Moreover, the health systems in these countries were unable to escape many of the criticisms which were valid for systems in the 'First World'. The conclusion of such a flood of criticism was the need to *move away from the hospital-centred and specialist-centred model*, which remained dominant until then, and to create the type of health-care model and mechanisms known as *Primary Health Care* as from the Alma-Ata conference (WHO, 1978, 1992, and Tables 1-3).

*Table 1.* Conceptual elements of primary health care

| CONCEPTUAL ELEMENTS OF PRIMARY HEALTH CARE |
|---|
| • Comprehensive<br>• Integrated<br>• Continuous<br>• Permanent<br>• Active<br>• Accessible<br>• Interdisciplinary and bio-psychosocial teams<br>• Community-based and participative<br>• Programmable-assessable (able to evaluate).<br>• With teaching and research |

But as *Primary Health Care* began to be applied and set into operation, with the intention of putting the proposed features of the model into practice, problems began to appear (WHO, 1992; González y Levav, 1991; Martín, 2000; Tizón, 2000). The first of these, a ceaseless increase in the demand (and, in some cases, the frequentation) which the *Health Centres* had to bear in every location (from the first- to the fourth-worlds). Another problem which arose was that a significant number of the visits to these centres were... because of mental health problems (25-30%: Goldberg and Huxley, 1980, 1992) or because of «biologically inexplicable complaints» (more than 10%) (Tizón, 1992, 1997; Epstein, 1993, 1996). This has led to the need for contacts, joint consultation and efforts at shared work, between family doctors/GPs or paediatricians on the one side, and mental health staff on the other. Significant difficulties soon appeared regarding this co-operation (WHO, 1992; Tizón, 1992, 1996). From this standpoint a complementary line of health care has had to be developed, which some have called *Primary Mental Health Care* (Tizón, 1990, 1992, 1996, 1997, 2000).

*Table 2.* Characteristics of primary health care

| **Characteristics of Primary Health Care**<br>(from the psychosocial point of view) |
|---|
| 1. Moving health care closer to the population. |
| 2. Integrating it into territorial and individualised teams. |
| 3. Diachronic perspective. |
| 4. Theoretical, technical and biopsychosocial model |
| 5. Integrating prevention-promotion and care (= **"Attention"**) |
| 6. Not opposed to "lay" or "non-professional" systems (but improves their efficacy, effectiveness and efficiency). |
| 7. Should it avoid making the "professional health systems" indispensable. |
| 8. Therefore pays special attention to<br>Iatrogeny }<br>iatrogenic chronicity } = heteronomise<br>medicalised chronicity } |
| therefore, **CENTRIPETAL WITH REGARD TO THE COMMUNITY**<br>(=usual experiential groups or nucleus) |

A third problem arising from the first years in which PHC has been running has to do with the very aims of the reform. To aim for a wide-ranging «bio-psychosocial» view of the patient; to encourage the professional to achieve an overall perspective (Table 3) implies, of course, a significant increase in the anxieties and conflicts facing that professional.

*Table 3.* The change which the development of PHC involves

| | TRADITIONAL MEDICINE | PRIMARY HEALTH CARE |
|---|---|---|
| AIMS | Illness | Health and Illness |
| | Healing | Prevention and care |
| CONTENT | Treatment | Health promotion |
| | Occasional care | Continuing care |
| | Specific problems | Comprehensive care |
| ORGANISATION | Specialists | General practitioners |
| | Doctors | Inter-professional |
| | Individual practice | Teamwork |
| RESPONSIBILITY | Health sector | Inter-sector co-operation |
| | In isolation | Community participation |
| | Professional control | Self- responsibilisation |
| | Passive reception | Prevention in General Population |
| FOCALISATION | Biological | Bio-psychosocial |

As well as trying to keep up-to-date with the biological techniques of medicine, PHC professionals must also, by obligation, improve their psychological and psychosocial techniques and capabilities. All this at a time when the professional feels more personally «committed» to the patient-doctor relationship (and in each relationship with each patient) than does his/her hospital-based counterparts. Resulting from this significant increase of anxiety among the professionals of the said health centres is a generalised state of worry, which often takes on a «reparatory» aspect («depressive» in the sense of M. Klein), but which in other cases is overcome by persecutory or confusional experiences and anxieties (Bofill and Tizón, 1994; Tizón, 1996).

This is one of the paramount reasons why psychoanalysis, and the psychoanalyst who is appropriately interested, trained and integrated in PHC psychoanalysis, can be so useful for the development of PHC. Psychoanalysis (some psychoanalysts) could co-operate with - and may co-operate within - PHC in the following five basic ways:

1. Giving support for personal development, work setting, professional training and group- or team- organisation for many of those who work in health centres: a *clinical-preventive and developmental contribution* to PHC.
2. Offering elements for the practical-theoretical and epistemological basis upon which to lay the fundamental principles of PHC: *a theoretical contribution.*
3. Offering psychotherapeutic elements, which can be used by primary health care professionals and mental health teams: *technical contribution.*
4. Offering a number of *pragmatic elements* both to PHC and mental health teams.
5. Offering elements of the previous four types for a renewed practice of *Community Mental Health Care* (the *Primary Mental Health Care* model: (Tizón, 1992, 2000).

## 2. PSYCHOANALYSIS AND PRIMARY MENTAL HEALTH CARE (PMHC)

We use the term *Primary Mental Health Care* to describe the application of the «patient centred care» model (Balint, 1968, 1973) or «care centred on the consultant» model (Tizón, 1981; Borrell, 1986; Epstein *et al.*, 1993; Stewart, 1995; Tizón, 1992, 1995, 2000) for the interdisciplinary work of mental health care in the community, supporting the primary health care team. This way of attending to (prevention and treatment in) health and (mental) health will possess, in brief, a number of basic features which I have spent over twenty years promoting:

1. A theoretical link with the PHC model.
2. A practical link and strong connection with the actual PHC centres: this line of work implies that mental health problems, as well as prevention work in this field, must be the shared responsibility of both PHC staff (GPs and paediatricians) on one hand and by community mental health staff on the other.
3. Both types of staff should, moreover, be sufficiently interlinked with the rest of the professional care networks in their field: social services, psycho-pedagogical services, psychosocial services of legal and justice systems, community social welfare systems...
4. They will have to share the workload with the «lay» networks or non-professional social network: local groups belonging to the resident population; NGOs; sport or recreational groups *etc*.

Primary (Mental) Health Care would be, then a way of providing community mental health care and psychiatric care with the support of PHC staff, in particular, and with the combined aims of: i) improving the capacity of PHC staff to deal with problems of «mental health» and ii) to encourage a progressive exchange of knowledge, techniques and skills between both types of staff.

## 3. THEORETICAL ISSUES

I shall continue, in this section, with the classic subdivision of the domains of all scientific disciplines: theoretical, technical and practical – to which should be added an epistemological view, though I cannot enter into this here. As I understand it, the basic theoretical applications of psychoanalysis to a not-strictly-psychoanalytical clinical practice tend to be based on the following features: a) several general meta-theoretical principles; b) an explanatory model of mental disorders and their origins (for example, the one exposed in Table 4); c) a model for the interaction of the biological, the psychological and the social (a certain conception of the bio-psychosocial model: Engel, 1977); and therefore d) a frame of reference to explain numerous phenomena associated with illness and with the experience of becoming ill (and seeking care).

At a theoretical level this implies that it would be difficult to speak of «Primary Care» in the case of health care which did *not* take into account, on the one hand the internal world, the world of mental representations (emotional, cognitive ...), and on the other the micro social group, the family, and their mental representations. And I believe that this care model should take these elements into account with the explicit and deliberate purpose of preventing psychosocial conflicts from becoming chronic: the mental disorder, illness or disability... Here we find the role which psychoanalysis - as a frame of reference, and as «psychological theory» (or *meta-psychology*, in Freud's sense) – can play in Primary Health Care. It can represent one of the possible psychological frames of reference for understanding the internal world, its relationships with the external world and the role of both in the processes of generating psychological conflicts and of these becoming chronic conflict («chronification» is the basis of mental disorders).

*Table 4.* Paramount preventive notions in mental health

| | | |
|---|---|---|
| **RISK FACTORS**<br>(Internal/external) | **INNATE DISPOSITIONS**<br>+<br>**INITIAL RELATIONSHIPS and CONTINGENCIES**<br>+ | **CONTAINING FACTORS And RESILIENCE Levels:** |
| **VULNERABILITY**<br>of - social<br>- family<br>- individual<br>- and mental<br>SYSTEMS | **BIOLOGICAL, PSYCHOLOGICAL and SUBSEQUENT SOCIAL CONTINGENCIES** | 1. From the object internal world<br>2. Ego capacities<br>3. Body & "body self"<br>4. Family<br>5. "Lay" networks<br>6. Professionalised networks |

⇩

WARNING SIGNALS
Biological
Psychological
Social

⇩

PSYCHOPATHOLOGY and/or MARGINATION
* in childhood
* afterwards

**TERTIARY PREVENTION**
Rehabilitation and reinsertion

**SECONDARY PREVENTION**
Early detection and treatment

**PRIMARY PREVENTION** **PROMOTION OF MENTAL HEALTH**
Avoid the appearance of the disorder

With regard to models of interaction between the biological, psychological and sociological conditioning factors of mental disorders, psychoanalysis will concentrate on the study of psychological conditioning factors and, even more, on the study of intra-psychic and relationship factors. These include: the background of the first human relationships and personal risk factors – with special attention to emotions, mental suffering, and to how the patient lives with these: their motivation and personal standpoints – «programming» the basic guidelines for relating to others (object relationships), *etc.* (Table 4). All this would not be exclusively by way of experimental methods or retrospective searching, but rather by the study of transference and counter-transference, from the affective movements perceived in the here-and-now of the consultation.

On a technical and pragmatic level, the above applications may be specified, as we have seen, in the following situations or day-to-day areas of work:

1. Area of observation and attention.
2. Area of diagnosis and intervention.
3. Area of teamwork and internal co-ordination.
4. Area of co-ordination with the exterior.
5. Area of training.
6. Area of research.

In this particular field of Primary Health Care, I believe that psychoanalysis provides, or could provide, at least the following elements:

1. Regarding the first area or the field of day-to-day work, psychoanalysis can provide, as well as the theoretical aspects already mentioned, some indications about the essential care tool: the clinical interview, which may not be overlooked. In reality, psychoanalysis and its various applications provide, above all, elements for individual - family or group interviews, which comprise the most often used technique in PHC (the only one necessary in one hundred per cent of consultations).
2. Adding this fact to the theoretical framework of PHC and of contemporary health care, I believe that the main applications of psychoanalysis in primary care approach implies something similar to the bio-psychosocial model with psychoanalytical or «relational» basis (Tizón, 1988, 1992, 2000; Stewart, 1995). In this sense the applications and psychoanalytical supervisions would have to be orientated above all towards helping to maintain the internal setting of professionals with different backgrounds and training, as well as the team as a whole. Especially, it should help them to maintain three indispensable perspectives: overall vision, ideological neutrality and emotional containment. *Overall vision*, in the sense of helping them to maintain an overall, integrating and bio-psychosocial perspective of the patient, not forgetting the internal world of the health care seeker (his/her internal objects, affects, sentiments, cognitions...). *Ideological neutrality* and *emotional containment* in the sense of personal neutrality towards the

patient, much more important in primary care settings, where staff are constantly under pressure to be «flexible» regarding technical modifications or the use of various new techniques – a notion so easy to confuse with compliance and collusion.

3. Another set of contributions that psychoanalysis can offer PHC in this area regards the different ways and motivations of making a health-care consultation, and about the bio-psychosocial experience of becoming ill («the illness experience», Balint, 1968, 1973; Stewart, 1995). In the same sense, it can improve and broaden the capacity for observation and the observation techniques relevant to care. In particular, from a pathognomonic view of psychoanalysis: the observation of the relationship and counter-transference which this itself sets in motion (on PHC settings I have called this «to observe and to observe oneself observing»).
4. In the area of diagnosis, psychoanalysis provides considerable data concerning types of relationship, lifestyles, psychopathology, conditioning «psychosomatic» relationships as well as understanding mental disorders, conflicts, suffering and fundamental psychosocial transitions. But, in this field, to be able to work together with PHC, we psychoanalysts must be able to distance ourselves from our own mythologies and narcissism as a group, for example, in the «psychosomatic» field (Tizón, 2000).
5. At a diagnostic and therapeutic level we should not forget an outstanding fact regarding current health care practice: that more and more health care services tend towards the subdivision of the human individual, towards *a partial object care*. Psychiatry, too, more and more treats the human being as a set of «partial objects» (*i.e.* neurotransmitters) within that «production line of manufacture, reparation (and assembly)», in which every health worker applies his drug, his partial intervention, or puts another screw in place. At least as a model, PHC is the type of health service outlet most different from this dominant trend, made worse by economic interests and economicism. Therefore, more and more often, it is the family doctor or paediatrician who asks what is happening with the patient who has been taking «new generation» antidepressants for three, four or five years – how is his or her overall health; and, should another type of approach be tried? Or: what will happen to the child to whom somebody has recommended taking stimulants for the central nervous system over three, four or five years – since childhood! - because of a supposed «disorder of attention deficit with hyperactivity»?

## 4. TECHNICAL AND PRAGMATIC LEVELS

1. At the level of therapeutic techniques we should remember for instance the «flash» psychotherapies and «flash» techniques or techniques of sensitisation «to the psychological» (Balint, 1968; Tizón, 1997); the psychological aid available from PHC itself (for disorders of anxiety and depression for example); «orientation or counselling with a psychodynamic basis»; «promoting health and preventive rules of behaviour» from the psychodynamic perspective (in childhood and adulthood); «contention interviews»; interviews and processes for the management of grief; group therapies applicable within PHC, *etc.*
2. Furthermore, we should remember the actual availability of clinical guides for PHC services with a psychoanalytical basis such as: care for

*Table 5.* Group therapies carried out with PHC-PMHC shared working

**(Direct) CARE GROUPS**

- **Alcoholics**
- **Alcoholics** and relatives
- **Mutual Aid** and socialisation
- **Dysthymic** patients
- **Drugs**: Group of relatives of the **drug-dependent subjects**
- **Pregnant** and lactating women
- **Neurological**: Group of relatives of patients severely affected by neurological diseases
- **Severely ill**: Groups of relatives of severely ill or chronic patients
- **Family:** Family interviews
- **Migrations**: Group on **migration** and mental health
- **Middle-aged Women's Group**
- **Parallel**: (Parallel) group of relatives of **children** who attend groups (or periodic therapies)
- **Psychotic**: Group of relatives of psychotic patients
- **Relaxation**
- **Somatisers and heavy consumers of health care**

**GROUPS INCLUDED AMONG PREVENTIVE PROGRAMMES**

- **Psychological aid to maternity:** Pregnant and lactating groups
- **Parents**
- **Neuroleptic retard group**
- **Obesity – weight control**

**GROUPS WITH CARE STAFF:** Groups of:

- **Interconsultation**: (the interconsultation as a group)
- **Reflection with nursing staff** from the health centre
- **Reflection** on **health care and administrative problems** with staff from medical inspection and management
- **Reflection on psychological problems** for "non-medical" staff in health care
- Reflection on **parent-child relationships** with paediatric staff
- **Theoretical seminars** as with "working groups"
- **"Balint-type" groups** or groups of reflection on the relationship problems of health care practice
- **Functional Unit for Mental Health Care** of early infancy

agoraphobics; contention; withdrawal from psychopharmacologic products; psychodiagnostic elements for PHC; family interviews; interviews with accompanied patients; problems with a partner; use of psychopharmacologic drugs in relation to basic anxieties; relational relaxation; approaches to patients with somatomorphic complaints; follow-up of «open to flash», *etc.* (Tizón, San José, and Nadal, 1997, 2000). Also some group therapies, such as those shown in Table 5: these are techniques which we have already put into practice with some PHC teams, working together with PMHC staff – such as the care programs for children shown in Table 6.

*Table 6.* Health care programmes for primary mental health care in children

| TRADITIONAL | ADAPTED |
|---|---|
| | Protocol type |
| Elementary group techniques | Problems with **meals** |
| | Functional **enuresis** in childhood |
| Scenotherapeutic techniques | **Language and speech** disorders in childhood and adolescence |
| Psychoanalytic help to families | **Day-to-day incompatibilities** between parents and children |
| Cognitive-behavioural help for families | **Follow-up** of children with **neurological** risk-factors |
| Interconsultation with paediatrician (Consulting liaison group) | **Follow-up** of children with high risk of mental disorder |
| | Childhood **sleep disorders** |
| "Balint-type" group with paediatric staff | |
| | Group programs |
| | **Asthmatic**: groups of parents of severely affected asthmatic children |
| | **Self-expression** and play for children of six years and above |
| | **Parallel group** for families of children who attend groups (or periodic therapies) |
| | **Group of parents of enuretic children** |
| | Reflection group on parent-child relationships with paediatric staff |
| | Others |
| | Relationship-based psychomotricity and logopedics |
| | Relationship-based re-education and psychopedagogy |

1. In the areas of teamwork and co-ordination, psychoanalysis offers various techniques and ways of working in groups: supervision; discussion groups; groups for reflection; operative groups; «Balint-type» groups, *etc.* (Tizón, 1992, 1993, 1998). To date we have been running

«Balint-type» groups for over twenty years in particularly conflictive and/or scientific-biased (scientificist) care settings. Some such groups are now at the stage of their 13th year stage.

2. In the area of training, there is a fundamental contribution from psychoanalysis, which is that of supervision or tutorials in the care setting, both individual and in groups. This method, with or without the psychoanalytical frame, has been acclaimed by all types of training experts. In Catalonia, with the experience we have accumulated, we have even managed, with the help of our psychoanalytical perspective, to define a minimum programme and a prioritised programme for the continuous training in mental health of members of PHC staff throughout Catalonia, paying special attention to prevention (Tables 7 and 8). In general, in this field of training, the application of psychoanalysis stresses the importance of «learning through experience» and the value of shared emotions as a fundamental form of teaching for clinical practice, for (general) health or for mental health.

*Table 7.* The Generalitat of Catalonia's priority programme for continuous training in mental health for primary health care.

| PHC PAEDIATRICS | FAMILY & COMMUNITY MEDICINE | NURSING | SOCIAL WORK |
|---|---|---|---|
| 1. Course of clinical interview | | | |
| 2. Basic training course in mental health for PHC | | | |
| 3. Introduction to FAMILY care from PHC | 3. Introduction to FAMILY care from PHC | 3. Psychological aspects of NURSING CARE | 3.Intervention of social work with specific groups of patients |
| 4. PREVENTIVE PROGRAMMES for PHC paediatrics | 4. Approach to BEREAVEMENT AND LOSS | 4. Psychosocial intervention of nurse (level II). | 4. Group techniques for PHC social work |
| 5.(BALINT-type) reflection groups // or Seminars on basic anthropology | 5. Early detection and treatment of DEPRESSION // or (BALINT-type) reflection groups | 5. (BALINT-type) reflection groups | 5. (BALINT-type) reflection groups |

Adapted from the Advisory Council on Mental Health in Catalonia, 1996

1. As for research, the influence of psychoanalysis can be seen in the importance attached to clinical investigations, to careful attention to the clinical setting in investigations, to broad and contextualised

perspectives in such investigations, and to the emphasis on respect for the patient and the ethical norms of the research. Regarding specific information, in our unit we are currently undertaking research along the following lines: Mixed therapeutic systems (psychoanalytical-cognitive); the value for health care of a «psychologically based psychiatry» - at a time of uncontrolled biological bias (biologism) within the system; also about group techniques; preventive programmes in mental health; symptoms of mass hysteria or epidemic somatomorphic disorders; schizophrenia and its antecedents in childhood and in adolescence; warning signs of psychopathology in early infancy; preventive programmes during pregnancy and the puerperal period; the role of the father ...

*Table 8.* Mental health prevention programmes from PHC, the Programme for Preventive Activities and Health Promotion (PAPPS) of the SEMFYc*

| **PROGRAMME** | **Promotion and prevention activities for mental health in children, including** (or incorporating) from other programmes |
|---|---|
| **"HEALTHY CHILD" PROGRAMME (Paediatrics)** | *Follow-up of psychomotor development (Haizea-Llevant).<br>*Childhood and Adolescence Mental health protocol. |
| **PROGRAMMES of P.H.C. for CHILDHOOD and ADOLESCENCE (Family Medicine)** | *Ocular and sight-related abnormalities.<br>*Hypoacusia.<br>*Accidents in childhood.<br>*Maltreatments and negligence on child. |
| **MENTAL HEALTH PROGRAMME of P.A.P.P.S. (Family Medicine)** | *Care in pregnancy and lactation.<br>*Pregnancy in adolescence.<br>*Children of single-parent families.<br>*History of psychiatric pathology in parents.<br>*Failure in school.<br>*Disorders in the development of language.<br>***Activities in common with adults*****:**<br>*Prevention of suicide.<br>*Secondary prevention of depressive disorders.<br>*Secondary prevention of disorders due to excessive anxiety. |

SEMFYC: Spanish Society of Family and Community Medicine.
PAPPS: Program for Preventive Activities and Health Promotion of the SEMFYC
***With a lesser degree of application in childhood and adolescence than the rest of the programs and sub-programs.

1. As for prevention and health promotion, the only immediate examples I can show are the outlooks summarised in Tables 8 and 9.

*Table 9.* Preventive programmes for primary mental health care in early childhood for a mental health unit linked to PHC

| Belonging to PHC or shared work with MHU | Shared work PHC - MHU |
|---|---|
| | Coordinated by the Mental Health Teams (MHT) |
| * **Psychological and psychosocial assistance to maternity:** Groups of pregnant and puerperal women. | * **Psychological and psychosocial assistance to maternity (paternity).**<br>* **Balint-type groups with paediatricians, nurses, management staff,** ***etc.***<br>* **FUNCTIONAL UNIT FOR MENTAL HEALTH CARE** IN EARLY CHILDHOOD. |
| * Preventive-teaching group and programme "Nurseries and observation of babies" | * **Nurseries and observation of babies.**<br>* **Therapeutic observation in childhood.** |
| * Group of mothers and fathers. | * **Follow-up** of child with high risk for **mental disorders.**<br>* **"Sickly" children.** |
| * **Follow-up** of children with **neurological** and/or sensorial **risks** | * **Reflection groups** on **parent-child relationships** with paediatric staff.<br>* **"Theoretical" seminars** as far as working groups. |
| * Massage and relationship with baby | **MENTAL HEALTH PREVENTION PROGRAMMES OF THE SPANISH SOC. OF FAMILY DOCTORS (SEMFyC):** |
| *** Others | * Care of woman and baby in **pregnancy and lactation.**<br>* **Pregnancy in adolescence.**<br>* **Children of monoparental families.**<br>* History of **psychiatric pathology in parents.**<br>* **Failure in school.**<br>* **Disorders in the development of language.** |
| | **PREVENTIVE PROGRAMMES LINKED WITH THE HEAD OFFICE FOR PUBLIC HEALTH**<br>* **Risk** factors and warning signals in the various stages of childhood.<br>* **Prevention in mental health in the "Healthy Child" Programme.** |
| | **OTHERS**<br>* **Asthmatics:** Chronic asthmatic children.<br>* **Asthmatics:** Groups of relatives of asthmatic children.<br>* **Hospitalised and post- hospitalised children.** |

1. Finally, I would like to say a few words about a preventive, clinical system for the earliest stages of infancy encompassed by PHC. This is also one of our fields of clinical research and one of the European Programs for Prevention in Mental Health in Early Infancy (European Commission, 52): Our *Functional Unit for (mental health) Attention in Early Infancy*, was set up on the basis of psychoanalytic techniques such as discussion and consultation groups and the psychoanalytic observation of babies – with the E. Bick system, adapted for PHC work by J.L. Tizón (Tizón *et al.*, 1997; Delgado *et al.*, 1999). The unit is now seven years old. It is composed of two working groups: the Interconsultation Group, partly closed, and the Seminary (or group) for Therapeutic Observation in Early Infancy, closed. Both are inter-professional groups, composed of paediatricians, paediatric nurses, psychiatrists and psychologists, infant care staff, social workers, kindergarten workers, and training staff from various disciplines, *etc.* In the Interconsultation Group (or liaison group) they discuss and follow-up interdisciplinary treatments in the cases of children and families with risk-factors or where there is a manifest psychopathology, especially in the first years of the child's life. Table 9 shows the types of help that, up to today, we have been able to set in motion for these children and families at risk. In the observation group, observations are carried out at the homes of some such babies; observations which are discussed in the fortnightly seminars. The observations are valid, above all, for the contention of the group observed and, besides this, for the training of the care staff.

## 5. A CLINICAL EXAMPLE

An exemplary case of the activity of the Unit was that of Viçens, an 18 month-old boy, sent by his paediatrician because of the frequent visits of his mother: she came every other day complaining that the boy «never stops, never. He doesn't sleep at all and only cries». The paediatrician had not been able to ascertain the reasons for the child's condition and presented the case to the consulting liaison (interconsultation) group. It was decided to carry out an observation of between 8 and 12 sessions at the home, to which the family consented.

From the very first observations, the observer was able to express her concern about the vulnerability of Viçens. He *not only slept*, and did not cry so much, but furthermore, it was observed that he could be left to sleep out in the corridor, alone, after hitting himself for minutes at a time against a wall or doorframe or practicing other auto-sensorial stimuli. The mother, present at the house, seemed never to connect with the emotional suffering of the child, although she was able to carry out the «operational» aspects of his care. The father, present in some observations, seemed much more sensitive to and in contact with these emotional aspects. But in the house (and in the mind of the child) it seemed that there was a sinister or painful atmosphere, which was not easy to explain ... until the mother's sister, and later the mother herself, were able to do so. The father was off work, gravely ill and waiting for a cardiac transplant which never materialised. Neither the paediatricians, nor the family doctor, nor the health centre's nursing staff were aware of this fact. They were also not aware that the father had twice attempted to commit suicide and that all the family was overcome with death anxieties. Once again, the unrestrained crying of an infant, of Viçens, was able to explain a situation of intense anxiety about death, and depression, of an entire nuclear family, anxiety that until then had only become apparent through the indirect channel of the projective identification on the child. In this way, the work in the Unit, and with the family of Viçens, as with so much other psychoanalytically-informed work in PHC, is both an important and fundamental clinical aid and a channel for awareness, knowledge and prevention.

Knowledge of clinical work from another perspective, prevention and integrated clinical aid. Here again we have the fundamental contributions, which, in my opinion, psychoanalysis can offer PHC in our time.

## 6. CONCLUSIONS

This chapter begins with a presentation of the model of Primary Health Care (PHC) and its relevance to health in the $21^{st}$ Century. In particular it stresses the issues concerning its psychological and psychosocial repercussions.

Thereafter it develops some of the applications of psychoanalysis, both for PHC and, more specifically, in mental health care in PHC: the model of Primary Mental Health Care (PMHC).

Generally speaking, psychoanalysis is considered to contribute to PHC in five basic ways:

1. Giving support to many of those who work in health centres in terms of personal development, setting preservation, professional training and group organisation: Clinical-preventive and developmental contribution to PHC.
2. Offering elements for the practical-theoretical and epistemological basis, upon which the fundamental principles of PHC can be laid out: Theoretical contribution.

3. Offering psychotherapeutic elements, which can be used by primary health care professionals: Technical contribution.
4. Offering a number of pragmatic elements both to PHC and to Primary Mental Health Centres.
5. Offering elements of the previous four types for a renewed practice of Community Mental Health Care (the model of Primary Mental Health Care).

In short, psychoanalysis should contribute to PHC mainly with clinical perspectives, with theoretical knowledge which takes account of the internal world, and by supplying the basic frameworks for prevention and integrated clinical assistance.

**References**

Balint M, 1968, *El Médico, el paciente y la enfermedad*. Buenos Aires: Libros Básicos.

Balint E, Norell JS (comps)., 1973, *Seis minutos para el paciente*. Buenos Aires: Paidós.

Bofill P, Tizón JL., 1994, *¿Que es el psicoanàlisis?: Orígenes, temas e instituciones actuales*. Barcelona: Herder.

Borrell F., 1986, Manual de entrevista clínica. Barcelona: DOYMA.

Brogren PO., 1985, Promotion of Mental Health. Helsinki: Nordiska hälsovardshögskolan Socialdepartament.

Consell Assesor en Salut Mental de la Generalitat de Catalunya - JL Tizón (coord)., 1995, Treballs, conclusions i recomenacions dels Grups de Treball sobre "Col.laboració i Suport amb l'Atenció Primária". Barcelona: Servei Catalá de la Salut, Generalitat de Catalunya (5 tomos).

Consell Assesor en Salut Mental de la Generalitat de Catalunya - JL Tizón (coord)., 1996, Inform Final i Recomenacions del Grup de Treball sobre Formació en Salut Mental per a la Atenció Primária de Salut. Barcelona: Servei Catalá de la Salut, Generalitat de Catalunya.

Delgado M, de Muga ME, Torregrosa MJ, Garrell J, Tizón JL., 1998, Observació assisténcial á la Primera Infáncia: l'Unitat Funcional d'Atenció a la Salut Mental a la Primera Infáncia (UFAPI). En I.C.S. (ed.) L'Atenció Primária de l'Institut Catalá de la Salut: Lligant CAPS. Esplugues de Llobregat (Barcelona): Departament de Sanitat de la Generalitat- Servei Catalá de la Salut, Regió Sanitária de Costa de Ponent (pp.34-36).

Direcció General de Salut Pública - Amigó E. et al., 1999, Medicina preventiva en l'edat Pediátrica: Procol de Salut Mental. Barcelona: Direcció General de Salut Pública - Institut d'Estudis de la Salut. Barcelona: Departament de Sanitat i Seguretat Social de la Generalitat de Catalunya.

Engel GL., 1977, The Need for a New Medical Model: A challenge for Biomedicine. *Science* 196: 129-136.

Epstein RM., 1996, The patient-physician relationship. En MB Mengel y WL Molleman (eds.). Fundamentals of Clinical Practice: A textbook on the Patient, Doctor and Society. New York: Plenum Medical Books (pp. 105-132).

Epstein RM, Campbel TL, Cohen-Cole S, McWhinney IR, Smilkstein G., 1993, Perpsectives on Patient-Doctor Communication. *J Family Prac.*; 37: 377-388.

European Commission -Mental Health Europe- European Commission: Mental Health Promotion for Children up to 6 Years: Directory of Projects in the European Union.Bruselles: European Commission 2000.

Goldberg DP, Huxley P., 1980, *Mental Illness in the Community. Fathaway to Psychiatric Care.* Londres: Tavistock.
Goldberg DP, Huxley P., 1992, *Common Mental Disorders.* London: Routledge.
González R, Levav I., 1991, Reestructuración de la atención psiquiátrica: Bases concpetuales y guías para su implementación. Washington: Organización Panamericana de Salud OPS - OMS.
Illich I., 1975, Némesis médica: La expropiación de la salud. Barcelona: Barral.
Manzano J, Palacios F., 1993, Las terapias en psiquiatría infantil. Barcelona: Paidós.
Martín-Zurro, A, Cano JF (dir.)., 1994, *Atención Primaria.* Barcelona: Mosby - DOYMA.
Martín-Zurro A, Ledesma A, Sans A., 2000, El modelo de atención primaria de salud: balance y perspectivas. *Atención Primaria*, 25, 1: 100- 113.
Meissels SJ y Shonkoff JP (comps)., 1990, Handbook of Early Childhood Intervention. Cambridge: Press Syndic of the University of Cambridge.
Newton J., 1992, Preventing Mental Illness in Practice. London: Routledge.
OMS-WHO, Alma Ata 1978: La Atención Primaria de Salud. Ginebra: OMS 1978.
OMS-WHO, 1992, La introducción de un componente de salud mental en la atención primaria. Ginebra: OMS 1992.
Palacio-Espasa P., 1993, La Pratique Psychothérapique avec l'enfant. Paris: Bayard/Paidós.
Pérez-Sánchez, A., 1996, Prácticas psicoterapéuticas. Barcelona: Paidós.
Red de Centros Investigadores de la Sociedad Española de Medicina de Familia y Comunitaria: Subprograma de Prevención en Salud Mental. En: Programa de Actividades Preventivas y de Promoción de la Salud. Barcelona: Soc. Esp. de Med. de Fam. y Com. 1999, 2000.
Royal College of General Practitioners., 1981, Prevention of Psychiatric Disorders in General Practice. Londres: Royal College G.P.
Royal College of General Practitioners, Royal College of Psychiatrists., 1993, Shared care of patients with mental health problems. Londres:Royal College G.P..
SEMFyC y PAPPS., 1999, Curso a distancia de prevención en atención primaria. Barcelona: SEMFYC.
Stewart M. et al., 1995, Patient-Centered Medicine. London: SAGE.
Tizón JL., 1981, Nueve tesis sobre la organización de unos dispositivos comunitarios de la Salud Mental. *Revista Mensual/Monthly Review*, 4 (6-7): 39-55.
Tizón JL, 1988, "Aspectos psicológicos de la salud". En R. Casares y cols. *La Salut (en record de Jordi Gol i Gurina).* Barcelona: Llar del Llibre - Escola Universitaria de Treball Social (pp. 25-51).
Tizón JL., 1990, Atención Primaria y Psicoanàlisis. Barcelona: Paidós-Fundació Vidal i Barraquer.
Tizón, JL., 1991, La Observación Terapéutica del Niño junto con su Madre en la clínica infantil. *Clínica y Análisis Grupal*, 13,3: 417-443.
Tizón JL. (dir)., 1992, Salud Mental en Atención Primaria y Atención Primaria a la Salud Mental. Barcelona: DOYMA.
Tizón, JL., 1993, Una perspectiva de los "Grupos Balint": Los Grupos de Reflexión. *Revista de la Asoc. Psicoanalítica de Madrid*, 18: 37-63.
Tizón JL., 1993. Los "Grupos de Reflexión" en la Atención Primaria de Salud.(I y II). *Atención Primaria* 6: 309-314 y 7: 361-367.
Tizón JL., 1994, Las psicoterapias psicoanalíticas breves y las "terapias de flash": I. La evolución técnica de las Psicoterapias Breves. *Informaciones Psiquiátricas* 138,4: 358-368.
Tizón, JL, 1994,. Las psicoterapias psicoanalíticas breves y las "terapias de flash": II. Los "Procesos de Sensibilización a lo Psicológico", Terapias "de Flash" o Psicoterapias

ultrabreves. *Informaciones Psiquiátricas* 138,4: 369-392.
Tizón JL., 1995, Apuntes para una psicología basada en la relación. Barcelona: Biblária (5a ed.).
Tizón JL., 1995, Los nuevos modelos asistenciales en Medicina: Una visión a partir de algunos de sus fundamentos psicológicos y epistemológicos. *Revisiones en Salud Pública* 4: 57-83.
Tizón JL., 1996, Componentes psicológicos de la práctica médica: Una perspectiva desde la Atención Primaria. Barcelona: DOYMA 1988 (5a ed.: Biblária, Barcelona).
Tizón JL., 1996, Notas sobre investigación y formación en la atención a la salud mental en la infancia. Clínica y Análisis Grupal ; 72, 18: 255-269.
Tizón JL., 1996, Posibilidades, medios y sistemas de relación entre los Equipos de Salud Mental y los Equipos de Atención Primaria. En JF. Otero et al. *Transtornos Psiquiátricos y Atención Primaria.* Madrid: DOYMA (pp. 31-52).
Tizón JL., 1997,Cognitivismo, psicoanálisis, psicobiología (II): Cognitivismo y psicoanálisis en las técnicas de psicoterapia. *Rev. Psiquiatría Fac.Med. Barcelona* 4: 133-138.
Tizón JL., 1997, Cognitivismo, psicoanálisis, psicobiología (III). Una perspectiva hacia el futuro. *Rev. Psiquiatría Fac.Med.* Barcelona; 6: 163-176.
Tizón JL., 1999, Prevención de los trastornos de salud mental. En PAPPS y SEMFYC: Curso a distancia de prevención en atención primaria. Módulos 5,6 y 7. (pp. 5-31). Barcelona: SEMFyC.
Tizón JL., 2000, La atención primaria a la salud mental: una concreción de la atención sanitaria centrada en el consultante. *Atención Primaria,* 26,2: 111-119.
Tizón JL., 2000, El tratamiento de la relación fóbico-evitativa: Desde la Psico(pato)logía Psicoanalítica hasta la Atención Primaria a la Salud Mental. En Grupo de Psicoterapia analítica de Bilbao (GPAB) (ed.): Las Fobias. Bilbao: GPAB.
Tizón JL., 2000, Reflexiones sobre "la psicosomática" a partir de la clínica psicoanalítica. *Revista de Psicoanálisis de la Asoc. Psicoanalítica de Madrid* 32: 159-183.
Tizón JL, , San-José J, Nadal D. 1997, 2000 Protocolos y programas elementales para la atención primaria a la salud mental. Barcelona: Herder.
Vuori HV., 1983, Qué es la atención primaria de salud? *Atención Primaria*; 0:3-4.
Vuori HV., 1987, Atención Primaria de Salud en Europa: Problemas y soluciones. *Atención Primaria* 1: 1-10.

# Training General Practitioners in the Psychoanalytical Aspects of Mental Health

*Considering the Situation in Switzerland*

José Guimón
*Professor of Psychiatry; Swiss Psychoanalytical Society*

The field of teaching psychiatry in medicine is in full transformation and should be examined as a whole in the context of a global problem concerning undergraduate and postgraduate medical education. As most people suffering from mental disorders and symptoms will never be seen by a psychiatrist, emphasis should be stressed on the education of general practitioners and other health care-providers.

A thorough transformation of undergraduate training has taken place over the last five years at the Geneva University Medical School. This paper will first emphasise the need for dynamic training of non-psychiatric physicians. I will then describe the educational objectives of the Department of Psychiatry and the modifications that have been introduced in the undergraduate medical curriculum. The advantages and disadvantages inherent in this new system will then be discussed. I will end with the recommendation that general practitioners obtain a dynamic attitude to contain the mental suffering of their patients.

## 1. THE NEED FOR DYNAMIC TRAINING OF NON PSYCHIATRIC PHYSICIANS

Psychoanalysis, probably has a wider future in general medicine than in psychiatry and thus, medical education should include the teaching of the theory and practice of psychoanalysis. In fact, from the beginning of psychoanalysis, many authors have been interested in what was called at that time "psychosomatic medicine", stressing the importance of psychological factors in health care. However, it is only recently that objective data has been available on the huge prevalence of psychopathological disorders among the general population and especially among those persons seeking the services of general practitioners.

## 1.1 The High Prevalence of Psychiatric Disorders in General Medical Practice

Based on the "Epidemiological Catchment Area (ECA)" research data, at least 19.1% of the general population will present a DSMIII-R diagnosis over any given six-month period. However, as shown by epidemiological data only a small percentage of the population with mental disturbances seeks specialised psychiatric help. Between one-third and one-fifth of those persons consulting a general practitioner have psychiatric symptoms. The ability of general practitioners to identify these symptoms is insufficient (around 60%) and when detected, symptoms are generally treated with psychotropic medication (which is not always adequate) and vitamins.

General practitioners have to "contain" the overwhelming mental suffering of these individuals and they generally do so without having any specialised training. Balint's groups represent one of the only ways of adequately facing this enormous challenge in psychiatry, but have been neglected until now. Tizon's works (Tizón, 1993a, 1993b) are of utmost importance in this respect.

The ways mental health problems are approached in primary care services vary according to the countries concerned (Tizón, 1996) in the British model of «derivation», general practitioners (with a great capacity for «containment») are the first recourse of patients with psychological complaints and refer them to psychiatrists. The «substitution» model proposes that family doctors and other professional networks (educational, social services) or laypeople (support systems) take charge of care. Psychologists and psychiatrists provide temporary support to primary care physicians until they can be replaced by well-trained general practitioners. The third model is that of collaboration between general practitioners and psychiatrists, working in proximity but at different locations, which fosters the risk of becoming a model of derivation. In the fourth model, real «mental health in primary intervention», the mental health team works at the same location as the general practitioner.

Whatever the relationship between primary care medicine and psychiatry, it is likely that in the future general practitioners will act (as is already the case in some countries such as the Netherlands, the United Kingdom, *etc.*) as the gatekeepers of the system and will be the first recourse not only for physical complaints, but for psychological or social problems, unless they arise in an emergency situation. In this kind of system, the patient must be sent to the specialist by the general practitioner, only if really needed.

# 2. A NEW EDUCATIONAL PROGRAM IN GENEVA

## 2.1. The Previous Situation

Swiss physicians - especially general practitioners and internists - are very interested in psychiatry. Training in medical psychology is an important part of the education of medical students in most Swiss schools of medicine. In a study carried out by Uchtenhagen (1993) in Zurich, it emerged that the overwhelming majority of students considered psychiatry as an important field of training for non-psychiatric physicians. Thus, 75% of 3rd year students and 88% of 6th year students considered that psychiatry was important; 40% of them believe psychiatry to be as scientifically based as other medical disciplines.

Medical students surveyed in Geneva on their psychiatric training were relatively satisfied with their educational grounding in most of the areas they considered to be important.

On the other hand, an opinion poll carried out with general practitioners and internists practicing in the Canton of Geneva (de Saussure *et al.*, 1996) shows that an important number of them elect to undertake some additional voluntary training in psychiatry during their medical studies besides the compulsory one. More than half (51%) of general practitioners and more than one-third of internists had under- or postgraduate training. Likewise more than half of internists and general practitioners took part in training groups for psychological problems and interpersonal relations. Approximately 30% of those physicians were involved in discussion groups, either in presentations whose objective was to improve the diagnosis of certain illnesses or as part of Balint groups, or even in programs which included personal psychotherapies, or yet again in supervisions which are offered by societies such as the Psychosomatic Association of Paris.

The organisation of out patient health care in Geneva, which depends predominantly on the private system, does not favour the integration of Mental health as a part of primary care. During recent years, however, the Departments of Community Medicine and Geriatrics have been developing out-patient networks where psychiatry could be easily integrated. Likewise, certain group practices (composed of physicians with various specialisations, including psychiatrists) already exist in Switzerland and new HMOs are being created all over the country, including the presence of psychiatrists. A problem arising from this model of collaboration is that of asymmetrical relations between the psychiatrists and the generalists, in the sense that mental health professionals speak of «how to teach family doctors», whereas, in fact, they have a lot to learn from them. An additional difficulty emerges from the fact that some family doctors and paediatricians, who have little interest in mental health concerns, rarely take part in common activities.

Nevertheless, this type of practice will continue to be anecdotal in our country and the models of substitution-derivation will probably remain predominant. Consultations for specific illnesses, seminars, didactic presentations, *etc.* should be developed more systematically for groups of general practitioners and internists, directed by well-trained psychiatrists. This should form part of the continuous training of physicians that is being progressively introduced in Switzerland. Programs should also be developed for the public, targeting the detection and management of psychological problems in primary care.

## 2.2. The Educational Objectives

Educational objectives have to be described in psychiatry as in each of the other fundamental medical branches. Two complementary basic approaches have been set up for defining psychiatric educational objectives. On the one hand, the professors of the discipline can define educational objectives in «consensus meetings». On the other, opinion surveys can be made inquiring into the abilities and attitudes in the field of psychiatry that a general practitioner should have.

A new curriculum for undergraduate medical education has been developed in Geneva with emphasis on problem-resolution oriented, small-group discussions (Guimón, 2.000). In order to establish educational objectives, seven hundred out of 1,540 doctors working in Geneva answered a questionnaire (developed by Guimón, 1980) on doctors' opinions concerning the necessary psychological and psychiatric contents needed for undergraduate medical education (Goerg *et al.*, 1996; 1999).

Some differences were noted between the priorities identified by Swiss doctors and their North American and Spanish counterparts. Summing up, both doctors and students in Geneva agreed with their compatriots on the importance of the following main topics:

- Establishing an adequate doctor-patient relationship (ability to discuss problems with their patients, to be familiar with the dynamics of the doctor-patient relationship).
- The detection of the principal psychiatric problems, with their elements of risk (differential diagnosis, psychopharmacological, referral to the psychiatrist, risk of suicide and necessity for hospitalisation).

- The management of a set of complaints with psychosocial, somatic elements linked to stress, emotional aspects for patients with chronic or terminal illness, alcoholism, drug abuse, *etc.*, which imply a knowledge of the social resources from which the patient may benefit.

The importance accorded to dynamic aspects varied according to the specific medical discipline (Table 1): They were more valued amongst non-psychiatrists than psychiatrists, amongst primary-care physicians than other physicians, and amongst primary-care physicians who had received specific education in the psychiatric field (in the form of training in psychiatry, for instance) than amongst those who had not received it. The areas considered to be important were largely the same in North America (Johnson and Snibbe, 1975; Callen, 1980; Holmes *et al.*, 1990; Chatham-Showalter, 1993) and in Spain (Guimon *et al.*, 1980).

*Table 1.* Comparison of Different Categories of Physicians (T Student and significance)

| What knowledge and specific expertise in psychiatry should a non-psychiatric physician possess? | Physicians/ Psychiatrists | Primary care Other Physicians | Primary care with/without psychiatric training |
|---|---|---|---|
| Ability to dialogue with patients about their problems | 3.23 ** | 2.52* | 1.89 |
| Ability to establish a differentiated diagnosis of the principal psychiatric syndromes | .71 | 5.67*** | .74 |
| Knowledge of social resources the patient can use | 4.95*** | 2.42* | 1.07 |
| Psychodynamic knowledge sufficient to evaluate the patient's behaviour | 5.90*** | 2.12* | 1.03 |
| Ability to evaluate the risk of suicide or the necessity for psychiatric hospitalisation | .77 | 5.45*** | 2.01* |
| Knowledge of when and how to refer a patient to a psychiatrist | - 4.88*** | -.05 | 1.22 |
| Ability to carry out short-term psychotherapies | 6.15*** | 8.86*** | 4.25*** |
| Basic knowledge of most common psychiatric treatments | .30 | 6.86*** | 3.03** |
| Knowledge of normal personality development | 4.57*** | .58 | 2.80** |
| Basic knowledge of the theoretical principles of psychoanalysis | 2.16* | 1.33 | 3.89*** |
| Knowledge of most common psychiatric medication | .50 | 7.12*** | .99 |
| Ability to diagnose and treat persons with mental retardation | .39 | 3.92*** | .52 |
| Familiarity with behavioural modification techniques | 3.37** | 4.04*** | 3.33** |

| | | | |
|---|---|---|---|
| Knowledge of physical alterations concomitant to emotional stress | .47 | 4.43*** | .70 |
| Familiarity with the dynamics of the doctor-patient relationship | 1.78 | 4.17*** | 3.99*** |
| Knowledge of emotional aspects of patients with chronic or terminal illness | - 2.08* | 3.63*** | 3.48** |
| Familiarity with the most common psychological tests and their use | 7.28*** | 3.94*** | -1.02 |
| Knowledge of behavioural disorders in children and adolescents | .10 | .84 | .56 |
| Basic knowledge of alcoholism and drug abuse | .58 | 2.11* | 1.44 |
| Basic knowledge of latest breakthroughs in molecular biology and neuroimagery in relation to psychiatry | .55 | 2.90** | 1.55 |
| Ability to diagnose and treat problems in the couple or family | 6.42*** | 4.81*** | 1.87 |
| Knowledge of sexual problems and their treatment | 5.33*** | 3.26** | 2.03* |
| Knowledge of the normal and pathological process of mental ageing | .50 | 1.62 | 1.90 |

* p <.05
** p <.01
***p < .001

The importance given by the different groups of physicians to the psychodynamic aspects in the training of medical students was, on the other hand, parallel to the extent of psychological problems they detected among their patients. Thus, general practitioners detected a higher percentage than doctors with other specialties (43 % vs. 30 %, p < .001) and those general practitioners who had some special psychiatric training, more than those who did not (50% vs. 34 %, p < .001).

## 2.3. A New Educational Programme

Undergraduate psychiatric training in Geneva formerly included traditional lectures, divided between the 6-year pre-clinical and clinical periods. During the latter, students would visit psychiatric wards to take down case-histories and attend patient presentations made by the unit heads of clinics.

Even if the abovementioned priorities did not always coincide with those proposed by the professors of psychiatry, they were taken into account at the time of establishing the educational objectives. The fact that the students considered certain common problems to be insufficiently taught, moved us to concentrate the program on the disorders frequently encountered in general practice.

A classic, discipline- and lecture-based approach existing in our Medical School was replaced by a new educational model that has been put into practice during the last four years with the help of a newly created Unit of Development and Research in Medical Education (UDREM), directed by a newly appointed professor (Christine Vu). The aim of the new program was to integrate the teaching of basic, clinical and psycho-social sciences with an orientation towards community health care, through active self-directed learning based on an extended practice.

The first-year curriculum uses a classical approach based on lectures on topics in physics, chemistry, statistics, anatomy, biology, embryology, physiology, organisation of the central nervous system and a 28-hour introduction to psycho-social medicine.

The curriculum for the combined second and third years consists of 11 four-week learning units (among them one on the Biological Basis of Behaviour), four two-week learning units to foster multi-system integration and a 27-month Clinical Skills program in small groups. Students are also offered a thorough community-based learning experience.

The fourth and fifth years begin with 12-week small-group sessions, comprising topics on the main medical branches including psychiatry and designed to facilitate knowledge of the mechanisms underlying common clinical syndromes. This is followed by a one-year rotation of 11 practice-based clinical clerkships lasting eight, four or three weeks. The clerkship in psychiatry lasts four weeks and consists in problem solving, case-based sessions emphasising self-directed learning. A standard week includes four 2-hour sessions of case-based discussions, 17 hours of self-directed learning, three seminars on non-psychiatric topics, six hours of medical visits, two afternoons of patient admissions and daily morning rounds.

The sixth year consists of ten consecutive months of full-time activity in elective subjects.

## 2.4. Students Opinions on the New Educational Programme

The students show satisfaction with the clinical pertinence of what they learn in the basic medical sciences. The new small group and problem-based learning have encouraged the participation of many students who previously did not participate in the traditional curriculum. From the tutors point of view, the contacts between clinicians and basic scientists have been reinforced thus increasing interdisciplinary work and the understanding of patterns of interpersonal and group dynamics.

As an intermediate internal report of the faculty (Bader, 1999) outlined, the integration of the psychological and psycho-social aspects of the «vignettes» has been less successful than that of basic and clinical sciences in the second- and third-year curriculum. Even when problems contained aspects concerning psychological issues, the students and tutors tended to put the emphasis on basic medical sciences and clinical aspects, rather than on psychological or psycho-social issues. The explanation for this probably lies in the fact that the choice of vignettes for the pre-clinical period was carried out in a group discussion with the rest of the tutorial body of the other Departments and our educational objectives could not be adequately maintained. In fact, the representatives of the other medical branches insisted on our taking responsibility for the biological basis of behaviour to the exclusion of the psychological aspects of illness - which had been the main component of our prior teaching activities. The result was that very skilled teachers, more oriented towards the transmission of knowledge of patient-doctor interaction and the physical expression of emotional conflict, desisted from taking part in this teaching and were replaced by equally skilled teachers of psychiatric neurosciences but who did not, in fact, have the necessary expertise to assure the other set of objectives.

In the clinical period, students were very satisfied with the clinical exposure they had to the main psychiatric syndromes. However, we realised that they had in fact been exposed to syndromes they would rarely see in their general medical practice. Mild anxiety or depressive disorders and other frequent psychological disturbances were not prevalent in the population to which the students had access. This consideration is now being brought to bear on the need to expand the population with whom they will have contact, to medical rather than psychiatric populations, in the guise of psychiatrists having special skills in the detection and treatment of these kinds of mild, frequent syndromes.

## 3. THE NEED FOR GENERAL PRACTITIONERS TO ACQUIRE A DYNAMIC ATTITUDE

Training in classical clinical psychiatry is of little value for general practitioners. On the contrary psychoanalysis could play a most important role in the improvement of doctor-patient relationship, in understanding the improvement of the psychological concomitants of physical disturbances and in the management of patients' psychic pain. A fundamental issue in this psychodynamic education is to facilitate an element of «containment capacity» provided by general practitioners, family doctors, paediatricians, nurses, social workers and all kind of mental health teams working in non-professional or informal centres.

We refer here to containment (Bion, 1977; Winnicott, 1971), of course, as the ability to be faced with anxiety, to comprehend it and project it in a way which robs it of its negative power. In this sense, there is an «internal» containment (dealing with one's own object representations), a «micro-social» containment (the mother, the original family unit, the analyst) and an «external» containment (social networks).

The formal support systems, professionally set up by health care professionals (including primary care physicians) tend towards dissociation and corporatism, becoming increasingly self-specialised and thus distancing the patient from the community.

Informal support groups (social networks, gaming or sporting clubs, the clergy, *etc.*) can serve as containers until they are overcome by the complex interplay of projective and counter-projective identifications stemming from the relation with regressed patients.

Patients suffering from mental health problems who consult general practitioners, may have already experienced numerous losses and frustrations. By the time they make an appointment with the GP, their personal capacity for containment has decreased and they may already have succumbed to very primitive anxieties leading to different bodily dysfunctions. A «good enough doctor» (In Winnicot's sense) can serve as a sufficient container. Institutions can also assure some containment and a health organisation which does not provide containment will promote disintegrating effects.

The basic job of the mental health team in primary intervention consists in backing up the family doctor in de-contextualising the physical repercussions of conflicts in order to confront the patients with their inner and interpersonal problems. As Tizón states «Most often, our job consists in helping patients not to further inflict damage on themselves, something which administrators find hard to believe».

## 4. CONCLUSION

Mental disorders are a major problem in public health and they are not sufficiently treated. We must develop research and teaching programs which are better adapted to the medical students' public and for targeted care-providers in detecting and the managing psychological problems in primary care. We must develop research on the detection of these disorders, on their prevention and treatment and on the transformation of the structural organisation of health services.

Specifically undergraduate medical training must teach medical students how to master relational competence, and psychoanalysis is essential for the transmission of such knowledge and attitudes.

**References**

Bion, W. R. (1977). *New Directions in Psycho-Analysis*. London: Maresfield Reprints.

Callen KE. (1980) Psychiatric Education of Nonpsychiatrists: Is it Relevant to Medical *Practice Psychosomatics*; 21,1:43-54.

Chatham-Showalter PE, Silberman EK, Hales RE. (1993); Learning Priorities of Staff, Residents, and Students for a Third-Year Psychiatric Clerkship. *Academic Psychiatry* 17,1:21-4.

de Saussure, C.(1996), *Opinion des étudiants de la Faculté de médecine de l'Université de Genève sur les contenus psychologiques et psychiatriques dans la formation prégraduée.* Thèse No. 9808 présentée à la Faculté de médecine de l'Université de Genève

Goerg D., Fischer W., Zbinden, Guimón J. (1996): Opinions des médecins sur les contenus psychologiques et psychiatriques dans la formation médicale pré-graduée. *Médecine et Hygiène*, 54:1768-1772, 1996

Goerg D. de Saussure C., Guimón J., Objectives for the undergraduate teaching of psychiatry: survey of doctors and students. Medical Education, 33:639-647, 1999

Guimón J, Totorica K, Villasana A, Ozamis A. Estudio comparativo de las opiniones sobre los contenidos psicologicos y psiquiatricos que se deben incluir en el "curriculum" de la licenciatura en Medicina. Actas luso esp neurol psiquiatr cienc afines 1980;8,3:179-90

Guimón J.: "Crise d'identidé et formation des psychiatres". Schweizer Archiv für Neurologie und Psychiatrie 146. 137-141. 1995.

Guimón J.: Consequences of recent changes in research and practice for the identity of psychiatrists. Eur Psychiatry 12(2): 92-98, 1997

Guimón,J.: New Forms of Psychiatric Education: The Geneva Experience. The European Journal of Psychiatry 14(1): 52-60, 2000.

Holmes GA, Musher JS, Wright HH, Butterfield PT, Cole EA, Smith ME. How Recent Medical School Graduates Evaluate the Clinical Relevancy of Their Behavioral Science Curriculum. Academic Psychiatry 1990;14,1:17-20.

Johnson W, Snibbe J. The Selection of a Psychiatric Curriculum for Medical Students: Results of a Survey. Am J Psychiatry 1975;132,5:513-16.

Tizon, J., Salamero, M., de la Alama, E and Diez Munguira, J.M. (1985) Introducción al biologismo; implicaciones teoricas, repercisiones.

Tizón, JL., 1993a, Una perspectiva de los "Grupos Balint": Los Grupos de Reflexión. *Revista de la Asoc. Psicoanalítica de Madrid*, 18: 37-63.

Tizón JL., 1993b. Los "Grupos de Reflexión" en la Atención Primaria de Salud.(I y II). *Atención Primaria* 6: 309-314 y 7: 361-367.

Tizón JL., 1996, Posibilidades, medios y sistemas de relación entre los Equipos de Salud Mental y los Equipos de Atención Primaria. En JF. Otero *et al. Transtornos Psiquiátricos y Atención Primaria.* Madrid: DOYMA (pp. 31-52).

Uchtenhagenl, A., 1993, Das Image des Psychiatrie bei Medizinstudenten und studentinnen. *Bulletin des Médecins suisses* 74, 17:668-672.

Ustin, B., N. Sartorius, 1995, *Mental Illness in General Health Care. An International Study*, John Wiley and Sons, New York.

Winnicott, D. W. (1971). *Playing and Reality.* London: Tavistock.

# Who and What is Psychoanalysis For Today?[1]

André Haynal*, Georges Abraham, Antonio Andreoli, François Ladame, Thierry de Saussure, Elsa Schmid-Kitsikis, and Daniel Stern
** Hon. Professor of Psychiatry, University of Geneva; Swiss Psychoanalytical Society*

## 1. WHAT IS PSYCHOANALYSIS?

Psychoanalysis is based on the thesis that experiences, particularly those of childhood, will later influence not only our reactions and acts, but also our expectations and imagination.

At the end of the 19th and beginning of the 20th century, Freud developed this thesis in attempting to help people suffering from their past experiences, or their «reminiscences», particularly those linked to their past and present desires - whether people were conscious of these or not. He came to consider the notions of desire and the unconscious as central to our understanding of the human being in his affective, relational and emotional dimensions. He set up a situation in which these desires and non conscious contents could appear and find expression; this is the initial meaning of the word «psychoanalysis»: treatment in which the obscure elements of desire, the unconscious, or sexuality, can come to the surface and changes can be achieved. These experiences led Freud and thinkers who followed him to conceive the development of mental or psychological activity. Psychoanalytical theory is based on a guiding principle and includes a great deal of data, observations, ideas of possible descriptions, and conceivable interpretations. Therefore, within psychoanalysis - which is not a strictly empirical science, but a reflection based on a particular experience - there are different currents. Obviously there are certain key ideas, as in

[1] As this was a round table, the spoken language used has been maintained deliberately.

philosophy; but there are many different thinkers and types of interpretation, many directions in the evolution of psychoanalytical thinking. Moreover, there are different ways or perspectives involved in how we view or consider psychoanalysis, starting with the ways we look at our experience with our clients. The question as to what is true or false is replaced by that of understanding the other and, on the basis of this experience, of finding a way of apprehending the human being. Finally, psychoanalysis has discovered ways of understanding neuroses.

Someone in a situation where there are no solutions, feels that life is such that they can see no way out. For this experience to finally become positive, the psychoanalyst must listen in a certain way. He listens to the person's concrete situation, but at the same time, behind the concrete situation he tries to search for other links, other references, another world behind this concrete world. This other world, the psychological world which the psychoanalyst perceives through what the person says, creates a new opening - this other world which belongs to the patient's past and his feelings.

We might argue today that the people who consult today have varying forms of «depression». Freud devised a situation which allowed the patient to externalise, reflect, at an optimal distance in relation to the listener: this gave birth to what is known as the psychoanalytical cure. Beside this "setting" psychoanalytical approach is naturally available to anyone, whatever their situation, through what are called «applications» of psychoanalytical theory: in a group, in the treatment of children, in psychotherapy or in psychoanalysis itself.

## 2. IS THERE ANY DIFFERENCE BETWEEN PSYCHOANALYSIS AND ANALYTICAL PSYCHOTHERAPY?

If someone has plenty of time, with professional and personal circumstances providing stability over a number of years, psychoanalysis becomes possible; the situation is different for someone with only a short amount of time available. The same applies for the intensity of the encounter: that of virtually daily encounters in analysis or once or twice a week in psychotherapy. This framework already imposes a big difference.

Some people will not undertake psychoanalysis because of constraints: financial constraints, the seriousness of the problem, fear of the future, lack of time, the need to move elsewhere.... The psychoanalytical situation is one in which the intersubjective tension within the field of the relationship is of prime importance for both partners present. It involves taking account of one's own subjectivity, assuming it as such. But in psychotherapy which is inspired by psychoanalysis, and in the area of psychotherapy as practised in reality, one is immediately involved also in a contract aimed at examining the reality of the problems which surround us.

The analytical approach, while focusing on working on oneself, allows one to look at various problems: psychosomatic, sexual, psychiatric and others, and provide help for those who are suffering. These cases involve analytical psychotherapy, carried out by analysts, guided by a psychoanalytical approach.

As a final point, the attitude will differ depending on whether psychoanalysis or psychoanalytical psychotherapy is involved. The situation inevitably differs according to the framework we are working in. As an analyst, one can work in psychotherapy also on a deep level, with more demanding constraints and in conditions which differ from those of the classic psychoanalytical cure. At the same time, there is a difference, the two polarities do exist, and it is sometimes difficult to situate ourselves in terms of a continuum.

The effects of psychoanalysis and psychoanalytical therapy may converge, the processes may be similar. Common elements exist in terms of process, technical approaches; basic differences exist in terms of the framework. The psychoanalytical framework provides much better access to fantasies, which require a certain number of weekly sessions; the nature of the process retrieves the archaic aspect of psychological activity. The psychotherapeutic framework faced with the same personality organisation remains more «superficial».

## 3. WHAT IS THE AIM OF PSYCHOANALYSIS?

A story which went round Vienna in Freud's day describes two men who both start psychoanalysis; after a few years they meet up and one asks the other «Do you still have any symptoms?» And the other answers «yes, but I'm proud of them». He has accepted himself: that is the aim of psychoanalysis.

The psychoanalyst serves to treat people who ask for psychoanalysis. In fact its aim goes far beyond the cure and treatment of patients. It is helpful for people who deal with human beings, like those who work in the field of health. It is helpful in hospitals, not only psychiatric hospitals, but where suffering is present. The psychoanalytical approach helps all those who are confronted by suffering – the nursing staff can try to comprehend the suffering on a deeper level and to understand the patient not only as someone who carries an illness, but as a complete human being. It helps us, whoever we are, to avoid seeing the human being in a dull, mechanical, one dimensional way. The contribution made by psychoanalysis goes well beyond the process of curing a number of people through psychoanalysis. It is the only theory in the humanities which takes full account of the complexity of the human being.

It would be tempting to say that psychoanalysis serves no purpose in psychiatry, because the latter uses effective methods, its own criteria, and has developed medication with considerable symptomatic action. But, this is not entirely true. When attempts have been made – and people have tried over the last few years in several countries throughout the world – to apply a perfectly scientific, medical model, designed to be utterly rational, it ceases to be efficient or satisfactory.

All children of a certain age, according to certain characteristics, want to marry their Dad or their Mum. A certain reality emerges from observing children, which has interested psychoanalysis – again, by applying a particular type of approach and references to mythology, *i.e.* that of Freud; this is referred to as the Oedipus complex. Freud did not set out to impose certain structures of explanation, but psychoanalysis is nevertheless based on a certain number of very precise findings resulting from clinical and child observation.

How do you deal with your body, and, through it, your drives, your flesh? And what help is available, if not psychoanalysis? The technique was developed as an extension of the human body. The wheel, the hammer, then writing and now the computer are further extensions of activity, an improvement on the human body. But the improvement is now such that the human body and its environment seem no longer necessary. Soon we will no longer be asked occasionally to speak in events in a virtual form, but will spend more and more time doing so and the fear is that we will soon be called upon to inhabit these spiritual states, on a permanent basis *i.e.* that we will be called on to remain in these spiritual residences which we prize so greatly but for which we are so little prepared. Take what happens at the cinema. We are invaded by more and more films set in more or less desolate surroundings, and the body is relentlessly attacked. You've seen «Fight Club», you've seen Kronenberg's films: the body is relentlessly destroyed, broken, in a kind of helplessness and we don't even suffer from this; you go back to the office the next day, mutilated *etc.* and at the same time, you go out into the streets, everyone follows along behind and the body is homosexually transformed, transsexualised, enhanced by all kinds of prosthetic devices; traumatology on one hand, and genetics *etc.* end up by showing us a new man who's practically immortal. So what are you going to do with your body? It will become a terrible weight, because you will have to get out of your body and come back to it, which is the most awful thing. Because all the scars you have will hurt at that moment. So there's a kind of moulting, modern man is like an insect ready to moult but he can't manage it. There is no simple solution: either he transforms the virtual into the artificial, into a reality which is totally artificial, or faces the solution we're all aware of *i.e.* nihilism, the hordes, nomadism on the net.

## 4. CAN EVERYONE BENEFIT FROM PSYCHOANALYSIS?

It is obviously hard to know, in the preliminary interviews, whether such and such a person, in view of their psychological makeup, capacity for insight and expression *etc.* will really be able to benefit from a long, costly undertaking which requires a lot of investment in time and money...Certainly not everyone...

## 5. WHAT IS THE TRAINING PROCESS FOR BECOMING A PSYCHOANALYST?

As regards training as a psychoanalyst, in many parts of the world, training is governed by strict rules. In many European countries, such as Switzerland, things are more flexible, without necessarily being any simpler. The essential first step is one's own psychoanalysis. Training is later carried out in stages lasting several years and approved by one's peers.

## 6. CONCLUSION

To conclude: the preceding remarks are a reflection of the discussions which took place: questions were asked; some of these remain suspended. Rather like in psychoanalysis...

# The Paradoxes of Seeking 'Psychoanalytic' Help for Private Matters in Public Places

Brian Martindale
*Psychoanalyst and Consultant Psychiatrist in Psychotherapy; Associate Member of British Psychoanalytical Society*

## 1. A CHALLENGE FOR THE FUTURE: SEEKING PSYCHOANALYTIC HELP FOR PRIVATE MATTERS IN PUBLIC PLACES

Psychoanalysis is more than a century old. In some ways it has penetrated every nook and cranny of our Western European cultures but the nature of the human mind is such that what is acknowledged can also be disavowed.

What I would like to do in this paper is to lay bare the enormous challenge that lies before psychoanalysis in the mental health field and to indicate that in this area of its application it has barely scratched the surface.

In our psychoanalytic training in the United Kingdom, a period of observation plays a vital part. Although it involves observing infants in their family homes, one purpose of this period of training is that it leads to the development of the capacity to emotionally take in and absorb without being able to relieve oneself through interpretation or other acts. I hope that what follows will make an impact on the reader and allow thoughtful reflection on the task in front of us.

# 2. PSYCHOLOGICAL DISTRESS IN THE 'PROVIDERS' IN THE HEALTH SERVICES

In a survey of psychological morbidity in doctors in five UK teaching hospitals, 25% of all consultants had measures of psychological distress that rated them as having a psychiatric disorder on well established scales (Kapur *et al.*, 1998). Other studies have indicated greater exhaustion and depression and suicide in psychiatrists than other specialities in spite of shorter working hours (Deary *et al.*, 1998; Rich and Pitts, 1980). Junior psychiatrists frequently suffer from depersonalisation in which they feel detached and uninvolved with their patients and unable to be empathic.

Within psychiatry in the UK in recent years, there has been a crisis of both recruitment and retention of consultant psychiatrists (Storer, 1997). Large numbers of consultant psychiatrists' posts remain unfilled. A survey published in 1997 by the then President of the Royal College of Psychiatrists found that 33% of those who retired before the obligatory age of 65 did so before the age of 55 (Kendall & Pearce, 1997). Early retirement contributed in a major way to many mental health teams operating without psychiatrists in key positions of leadership.

As psychoanalysts, we would all expect to find that the explanations for the distress and dissatisfaction of psychiatrists would be very complex, with a whole variety of personal and circumstantial components interacting. In this talk I intend to focus on one of the main underlying problems and its consequences for patient care.

## 2.1 Relationships and Mental Health Services

Because I suspect that it is relevant in other countries, I wish to comment as a psychoanalyst working in the UK mental health services. I will draw attention to the paradox of the genuine desire to provide quality mental health services and yet the lack of priority given to considering the *quality of relationships* as the crucial factor in this provision at all levels of the service.

This applies to:

- the treatment priorities for patients with mental disturbances,
- the training priorities of psychiatrists and the biological model of mental illness,
- the systems within which psychiatrists work in the public sector, the relationship with administration, management and government.

The following simple, simplistic, reductionistic, but complex and condensed statement that Winnicott attributes to fellow psychoanalyst John Rickman speaks to the mental guts of many of us psychoanalysts:

> *Mental illness consists in not being able to find anyone who can stand to be with you.* (Winnicott, 1985)

Rickman is pointing to the role of the social in generating mental illness. Lousada, with Winnicott and Rickman in mind, goes on to say that:

> *The question that must constantly be addressed in the modern welfare state (and, I would add, within mental health services especially) is whether there are people who can stand to be with those who cannot stand to be with themselves.* (Lousada, 2000).
>
> *[There is] an increasing state of mind in which recruits are scared of relationships, of feelings, of being too closely linked to their clients. Therapeutic benefit is linked to outcome and not to the relationship which provides the container for it.*

So what about relationships in psychiatry?

The decade of the brain has become plural – the decades of the brain. With all the hype about the genome project and the pace of technological advances there is increasingly no sign of any recovery of a balance in the predominant ethos practised in psychiatry in the UK. There is no sign of a return to an ethos in which the quality and understandings of internal and interpersonal relationships have a central importance – alongside understanding the brain, it's chemistry and neuropsychology and so on.

Leon Eisenberg, the distinguished emeritus Professor of Social Medicine and Psychiatry at Harvard, in a recent review for the World Psychiatric Association wrote:

> *Neuroscience is prospering, but the very pace and elegance of discovery in the neurosciences is reinforcing reductionism. The integration of brain science with mind science remains elusive.*

Fifteen years ago he had written his now famous quote:

> *Mindlessness in psychiatry was beginning to replace brainlessness.*

In his recent review he states:

> *Were I to be writing that paper today (his article of 15 years ago) I would be more generous in acknowledging the contribution of psychoanalysis..[Psychoanalysis] taught trainees to listen to patients,*

> *and to try to understand their distress, not simply to classify them.. etc. [Those] tasks are being squeezed out of clinical practice and residency training.*

So this brings us to the reason for the title of my paper. *The paradox of seeking 'Psychoanalytic' help for private matters in public places.*

I wish to emphasise the paradox that patients come to public services primarily for help with manifestations of disturbances in their internal and external relationships. These are matters of a highly personal and internally and externally 'unacceptable' nature – hence the disguises that we are all so familiar with.

The first paradox is that they are being increasingly treated by staff many of whom have very little focus in their training on understanding relationships, certainly little training in therapeutic relationships.

The second paradox is that according to the survey I have quoted, many of the psychiatric staff they see, in the UK at least, are themselves feeling helpless, hopeless and disillusioned about the quality of their professional lives and the relationships that they have with managers, administrators, and their psychiatric colleagues. The early retirement indicates a hopelessness of any benefit obtaining from their feelings being known and that relatively large numbers of psychiatrists are giving up their chosen career or planning to leave at the earliest opportunity that will be to their financial advantage. I am not suggesting that all psychiatrists who retire are mentally ill – but more to make the point that *they had no hope of relationships* in which their work problems and feelings and work relationship difficulties would be taken sufficiently seriously to elicit hope of good enough improvements. I want to make a close link here with Winnicott's aphorism quoted above.

## 2.2 A Typical Example – A Patient Comes for Help

I will next give an example of how a modern psychiatrist might think about a person who comes along with these sorts of problems as a patient – problems not dissimilar from the sort of problems that the psychiatrist is suffering from as a professional.

The modern psychiatrist, heavily influenced by the very seductive relationship with the pharmaceutical companies would be thinking that there is something disturbed in the patient's brain chemistry. The psychiatrist would listen carefully to his or her patient to determine what classification of disorder the patient has. The purpose of this is mainly to decide what medication will be offered. Follow-up appointments will be to see how the patient has responded to the medication and make adjustments. Certainly feelings will be elicited but the primary aim will be to decide what medication will best influence the feelings – usually to reduce their intensity. It will be quite unusual for patients not to be prescribed medication whatever their personal story.

To give an example: a 31-year-old man went to see a psychiatrist for the first time in a depressed state. His sleep was a bit disturbed and he was tense much of the time, but he was still able to interact at his work and in social settings. Because of his biological model of training, the psychiatrist prescribed antidepressants with a sedative effect to help improve his sleep and no other treatment.

Later when he did find his way to a psychotherapist, he told his story that in his 20s he had been living a certain life style, not too concerned about replacing personal and work relationships with others when they became unsatisfactory. From the age of 30 he had however become increasingly dissatisfied with this style of personal and work relationships but was feeling relatively hopeless and helpless at being able to influence the course of his future life for the better. From a psychoanalyst's viewpoint, the depression was a useful sign that something was wrong with his life and that he needed help with himself and his relationships. Aiming to relieve his depressive symptoms alone (with medication) might interfere with his motivation for help with the underlying problems.

The patient had however gone to the psychiatrist thinking that psychiatrists were the same as psychotherapists and would help him with his life problems. He could see that antidepressants might make him feel a bit better, but did not feel that it would be likely to do much better than the cannabis that he smoked at weekends. The cannabis gave him some relief from his worries about repeating the drifting lifestyle of his father, who died from the complications of alcohol which took over as his own relationships at work and in the family failed. The patient decided not to attend further appointments; one could say he retired or gave up on the health service.

## 3. THE PARADOX IN A NUTSHELL

I hope by now that you begin to get my point. The patient hoped for a relationship within which he could explore his difficulties in living a more productive life. It had taken him considerable strength to overcome his private feelings of shame and humiliation and to acknowledge his dissatisfaction with his life.

The paradox is that most psychiatrists would probably feel deeply offended if the range of feelings and hopelessness that they expressed about their work circumstances and its effect on them were to lead to them being told that the main way of resolving them was to take psychiatric medication.

So we have a very interesting and troubling situation; quite a deep split in which psychiatrists genuinely believe that medication is the primary answer for their patients' problems in living and are very sceptical about talking therapies let alone psychotherapies. The situation is even grosser with psychotic disorders. For example, in spite of overwhelming evidence over several decades that attention to the atmosphere of families with a psychotic member can dramatically affect relapse rate, few psychiatrists are trained in this way of working or allow their staff to practice this approach.

My main point that the malaise / disease discontent of psychiatrists is not too dissimilar from that of their patients. In the review by the College President mentioned above, respondents were offered an opportunity to voice their reasons for dissatisfaction. The vast majority of these reasons were related to the human conditions, burdens, expectations and relationships in which they were working. Retirement/ giving up working must surely reflect their despair about their feelings being attended to and taken sufficiently seriously. In essence they were reporting an overwhelming hopelessness about the human settings and relationships within which they were conducting their work and perhaps most importantly a hopelessness about being able to influence things for the better.

## 4. CONCLUSIONS

A longer paper would involve discussion about the ways in which psychoanalysts might be able to work in these circumstances with the collective states of mind, but to attempt this in this chapter would only dilute the impact of the disturbing state of health we find ourselves in. Suffice it to say that in the United Kingdom with its population of 55 million, the IPA society graduates about eight psychoanalysts each year and a similar number die. The challenge for psychoanalysis is an organisational one and not one of competing theoretical frameworks.

**References**


Deary, J.H. Agius, R. & Sadler, A., 1996b, Personality and stress in consultant psychiatrists. *International Journal of Social Psychiatry*, 42, 112-113.

Eisenberg, E., 2000, Psychiatry and neuroscience at the end of the century. *Current Opinion in Psychiatry*, 12: 629-632.

Kapur, N., Borrill, C. & Stride, C., 1998, Psychological Morbidity and job satisfaction in hospital consultants and junior house officers: multicentre, cross sectional survey. *British Medical Journal*; 17:511-12.

Kendell, R.E., & Pearce, A., 1997, Consultant Psychiatrists who retired prematurely in 1995 & 1996. *Psychiatric Bulletin*. 21: 741-745.

Lousada, J., 2000, The State of Mind we are in. *British Journal of Psychotherapy*. Vol 16, No 4, 467 -476.

Rich, C.L. & Pitts, F.N., 1980, Suicide by psychiatrists: a study by medial specialists among 18730 consecutive physician deaths during a five year period 1967-72. *Journal of Clinical Psychiatry*, 41, 261-263.

Storer, D. , 1997, Things have to get better. *Psychiatric Bulletin*, 21, 737-38.

Winnicott. D.W., 1985, *The maturational processes and the facilitating environment P218*. London. Hogarth Press and the Institute of Psychoanalysis.

# A Psychoanalytic Perspective on the Future of Mental Health
*Current Challenges*

Claudio Laks Eizirik
*Porto Alegre Psychoanalytical Society*

## 1. RECENT CHANGES IN MENTAL HEALTH

Thirty years of constant contact with the field of mental health, in its various forms and expressions, impel me to discuss some current challenges and future perspectives.

### 1.1 The Challenges of Biological Approaches

In this short period of time, historically speaking, I have witnessed and also participated in - sometimes adding impetus to - substantial changes in our field of activity: the exodus from the psychiatric macro-hospital and the advent of the general hospital; the idealisation of psychoanalytical techniques and of the explanatory power of psychoanalytical theories; the introduction and growing use of drugs; community psychiatry and its difficulties; the appearance of shorter and more specific psychotherapies; the improvement in diagnosis through successive multicentric studies; the appearance and improvement of research into psychiatry and into correlated basic areas; the appearance of post-graduate courses and their continuous expansion; the increasing specificity of psychoanalysis and its therapeutic effectiveness in relation to patients whose access is limited; the establishment of programs for the treatment of specific psychiatric disorders and the consequent increase in their therapeutic effectiveness; the idealisation of so-called biological psychiatry and of the explanatory power of the neurosciences; the growing presence and participation of the pharmaceutical industry in the daily life of psychiatrists and patients; the appearance of health-service provider companies and their interference in the privacy of the doctor-patient relationship; the changes in national health systems; the appearance of bioethics and their contribution to the study of the moral dilemmas in psychiatric, psychotherapeutic and psychoanalytical practice; the growing associative organisation of Brazilian and international psychiatry; more open discussions of questions such as the patient's rights, the multiple forms of sexuality, psychiatric internment; the expansion of liaison services; the increase of the interface between psychiatry and medicine, neurology, neurosciences; the decrease of the interface between psychiatry and psychology, psychoanalysis and the humanistic areas; the current emphasis on evidence-based medicine and psychiatry and studies on efficacy and the effectiveness of different treatments.

An inevitable consequence of these various changes is the acknowledgement that the very concept of mental health is suffering changes. Thus, one can identify different categories of «mental» and «subjective» well-being in Greek thought, in the feudal order, in modern thought and in the French Revolution, among others, each representing its respective historical moment, even if all of them remain operative in our culture (Stolkiner, 1988).

## 1.2 Psychoanalytic Approaches to Culture

Recent attempts to describe our culture from a psychoanalytical perspective derive from Freud's seminal contributions, while trying to underscore what is specific to the present time. What follows is a fragmentary summary of some of these attempts. (Eizirik, 1997).

Van der Leeuw (1980) characterised our Zeitgeist as constituted by (1) a great flood of information, quantification and massive growth that leads to superficiality, hampers independent thinking and is accompanied by a levelling process, as a consequence of which silence, solitude and privacy become endangered, and congestion disturbs man's consciousness of space and the experience of space he needs for his life; (2) changes in the role of the family as the basis of society, motherhood being increasingly neglected; (3) the dominant role of seductive advertising, encouraging immediate gratification and creating the illusion that total gratification is possible; (4) the increasing search for excitement, stimulation, brief and often violent explosions of emotions and the urge for rapid discharge, instead of the cultivation of warm, tender feelings, in particular where children are concerned.

From a wider perspective, Lasch (1978) coined for our era the expression «culture of narcissism», resulting from the breakdown of the family as a moral guidance system, the avoidance of conflicts by compromise and the accentuation of instinctive gratification. As social pressures have invaded the ego, it has become harder to grow up and to acquire maturity. This leads to a failure of normal superego development. So in a world dominated by images, individual progress can only come from projected images and erroneous impressions produced by insecure egos. In this world it is difficult to discriminate reality from fantasy, and what we really are from what the products we consume suggest that we are. The «culture of narcissism» has abolished collective discipline and concentrated work, in favour of a world of impressions, appearances and disguises.

Kernberg (1989) explored the nature of the appeal of mass culture, particularly as it is communicated by the mass media. He examined the regressive effects of group processes on the recipients of mass culture, and the striking correspondence between the conventional aspects of mass culture and the psychological characteristics of latency. Among others, he stressed the following trends in contemporary culture: the simultaneity of communication; the illusion of being a member of a crowd connected with a central figure who communicates what is important and what one should think about it; the denial of complexities; the predominance of conventional assumptions over individual thinking; the stimulation of a narcissistic dimension in the receiver, and also a paranoid one, in the form of justified suspicion or indignation; the application of a simplistic morality to social and political matters in the form of clichés (for instance, that good people together will solve problems). In his view, conventionality may be the price of social stability, in spite of the danger of more severe group regression. More recently, Kernberg (1998) described a striking tendency in large groups to project superego functions onto the group as a whole in an effort to prevent violence and protect ego identity by means of a shared ideology.

The postmodern condition, a term coined by Lyotard (1979) has become an essential part of any discussion of our culture. In spite of the controversial acceptance of this concept, several trends in our era are often described as typical of the so-called crisis of the culture: complexity, scepticism, challenges to all meta-narratives which were a central part of the project of enlightening, a crisis in the identificatory process due to a lack of self-representation of society as a shelter for meaning and values, acculturation through images in more and more virtual realities, claims to the right to difference and to following alternative lifestyles, the social demands for participation and for the rights of women, pacifists, homosexuals and other minorities, the growing presence of the so-called pathologies of immediate gratification, the idealisation of ambiguity, an era of simultaneity and immediate accomplishment of ideas, wishes and purposes (Arditi, 1988; Baladier, 1995; Castoriadis, 1996; Ahumada, 1997; Carlisky and Eskenazi, 2000).

This new culture which presents permanent change and complexity, produces increasing perplexity, schizo-paranoid and confusional anxieties, losses of models and values which are felt as a threat to the integrity of the self and a trend to internal dissociation. These are some characteristics of the men and women who will form the target population of mental health work.

## 2. PRESENT CHALLENGES

The mere statement of some of the recent developments in the field of mental hcalth, and of certain characteristics of our culture and of its unconscious repercussions, allow us to foresee what the challenges are. Confronting these challenges, and the possible consequences of this, will lead our activity in directions which tend to integrate or to disintegrate a field of knowledge and therapeutic action. I cannot establish a categorisation in terms of priority, *i.e.* the order of the challenges which I mention are not necessarily ranked according to importance, or vice-versa. However, I prefer to follow the path leading from the center to the periphery, from mental health itself to the training of its future practitioners and to their relation with the external world.

### 2.1 Mental Health and its Basic Sciences

Tension exists between the two main axes of thought in the mental health disciplines: the biological and the psychological. I do not include here the social axis because it does not seem to me that there is any major questioning of its relevance. The defenders of extreme biologism as well as the paladins of hardened psychologism admit that social factors play an important role, trying to attract it to their side. The real battle is between the explicative models, which are concentrated in psychoanalytical theories and those that derive from the neurosciences. I do not disregard the relevance of other psychological approaches either, but again this does not seem to involve such an obstinate confrontation.

The pendulum, at this turn of century, seems to swing powerfully toward the explicative power of the neurosciences, as in earlier decades it was psychoanalysis that was privileged. It is a difficult discussion because emotional aspects are at stake, and one should not disregard history, with all its traces of right and wrong, its exaggerations and arrogance. Former psychoanalytical arrogance has been replaced by the arrogance of biological psychiatry today. The present challenge, in my opinion, consists in recognising the complexity and multidetermination of normal and pathological mental phenomena. Any form of reductionism, besides being arrogant, is essentially incorrect, due to the limited explicative extent of only one theory to understand manifestations that are as complex as those we study and treat. The risk of a unidirectional view is its very tendency to allow the mechanisms of dissociation or fragmentation, which are found in the postmodern person, to also dominate the scientific sphere and to cause an impoverishment similar to the crisis in identificatory models already mentioned.

Thus, I think we should recognise the existence of certain basic sciences, such as those mentioned and others of a psychological, biological and social nature and to find the ways in which it would be possible to integrate them, or to develop and maintain a dialogue respecting the specificities of each. Two interesting examples related to this have recently appeared in *Molecular Psychiatry* and in the *International Journal of Psychoanalysis*. In the first, Nemeroff (1999) summarises and comments on the importance of studies which show that there is an increasingly impressive database concerning the long-term neurological consequences of untoward life events, *e.g.*, child abuse and neglect, loss of parents. Such alterations appear to increase vulnerability in several major psychiatric disorders, including affective and anxieties disorders. A case control study by Agid *et al.* (1999) provides further evidence for such an association, thus confirming Freud's theories about early traumatic effects on mental health and disease. In the second, we find a series of papers in the main psychoanalytical journal exploring the development of the neurosciences and their possible repercussions on psychoanalysis.

Another stimulating interface is constituted by the various studies on the effectiveness of psychoanalysis and analytical psychotherapy, summarised by Fonagy *et al.* (2000).

## 2.2 Psychiatry as a Medical Specialty

The fact that psychiatry is a medical specialty is common knowledge. The challenge of the moment is the disturbing impression that it is becoming so medical that it can lose its specificity. We went to the general hospital, integrated ourselves into medical schools, shared the same space and the same worries. But our patients are different and, necessarily, the way we approach and treat them is, too.

The doctor-patient relationship, which we have tried to teach and valorise so much, sometimes seems to be more learned and used by internists and paediatricians than by modern psychiatrists who are full of enthusiasm about technology and the therapeutic power of effective drugs, to the point of neglecting the person of the patient and of his or her family, with their internal worlds full of unconscious fantasies, expectations, fears and different anxieties.

Here, I want to characterise two common forms of reductionism, which we need to avoid: either that of ignoring the necessity of combined treatments and adopting an exclusively psychotherapeutic or psychoanalytical practice, in cases where the indication for medication is evident, or that of becoming a prescription-writer, ignoring the emotional experiences and psychotherapeutic needs - at least as a support - present in all patients.

The doctor-patient relationship - in psychiatry and any form of relationship concerning a mental health professional - is specific, complex and involves, more than in other areas, the emotional response of the therapist or his/her countertransference. How this therapeutic instrument can be used has been known, since ancient times and more precisely in the last century, thanks to psychoanalysis. However, recent progresses in the capacity of diagnosing and treating specific disorders in a purely manualised way may make us lose the ability family doctors had, and continue to have, of entering into emotional contact and, based on their own reaction, being able to identify what is happening with the patient.

In opposition to the current idealisation of objectivity, and of a practice highly based on scales, I would like to recall another way of visualising this concept: «Objectivity is based on a kind of internal dissociation that enables the doctor to partially identify himself with the patient and to take himself (his own subjectivity or countertransference), partially, as object of his continuous observation. This position allows him to be relatively 'objective' in relation to the patient» (Racker, 1957). The understanding of the meanings and uses of countertransference, and, in a wider way, of the analytical field (Baranger, 1961), enhanced the therapeutic possibilities in mental health, regardless of the form of intervention adopted. And this issue leads us to the problem of the training of future professionals of mental health.

## 2.3 Mental Health and Those who will Practice it in the Twenty-first Century

One of the most crucial and fascinating challenges of today refers to the kind of professional whom we think is best equipped for the next decades. If we consider complexity to be the trademark of our time, and that the natural trend points toward its intensification, the inference is that the future mental-health worker should be exposed to the widest possible range of learning experiences, kinds of patients and families, service «settings», theories and explicative models, and be able to practice his/her critical thought and creativity.

Right from the start of training, access to research and participation in research groups should be stimulated. Experience has taught us that identificatory models are the basis on which creative minds are built. This is a field in which the analytic training model reveals its usefulness very clearly, for it documents the possible ways in which to enable a professional to identify him- or herself with a mental function whereby listening to the unconscious and searching for the meanings of normal and pathological mental manifestations become his central *modus operandi*.

Thus, the future professional needs the experience of personal, private and sufficiently long contact with several supervisors, who will allow him/her to observe how they think and develop their clinical thinking. Supervision, with its style of workmanship, teaching and contact, and its mutual learning experience, is at the core of establishing a psychiatric identity. The challenge here consists in maintaining it and expanding its multiplying potential. I think that there is a current risk of teaching excessively or exclusively in groups, be it of theoretical studies or of supervision of the activity with patients. Without an experience of contact with the present day representative of the craft-master, the notion of the indispensable human relationship, which is at the basis of any mental health service, will hardly be established in the mind of the student.

The professional of the future will have to face new situations, some that are arising and others that we have only heard of. Just as examples, the increasing presence of elderly people in the population and their specific problems, the questions of bioethical dilemmas, the multiple forms of sexuality and the presence of service provider companies are some of the challenges we will have to learn to face together with our young colleagues. Models and formulas useful in the past decades cannot continue to be practiced and taught without periodic critical reviews.

Finally, one paradoxical question relates to the mental health professionals' quality of life. This area is one of increasing study and relevance to multicentric studies, although the fact that professionals who dedicate themselves to mental health often have a poor or difficult quality of life. Some time ago, it was almost unthinkable that a person in this field would not look for his/her own analysis or psychotherapy in order to be personally and professionally better equipped. This is one of the questions in need of attention, especially in the light of a prevailing model in which the basic requisite is that of efficiency and outcomes, relegating quality of life and its relation to mental health practice to a less important place.

## 2.4 Some Perspectives

If the present challenges I have tried to outline correspond approximately to the reality we are experiencing at the moment, its natural corollary is that some possible paths are offered to the mental health field, or different scenarios.

The first of them would be that of progressive super-specialisation and microspecificities, in such a way that we would have several psychiatries, psychologies, *etc*, linked to different approaches, each developing its way of understanding and practicing the specialty, leading to the fact that the very notion of something called psychiatry, psychology, *etc.*, without qualifiers, would lose its *raison d'être*. We would thus have total dissociation or fragmentation, with the constitution of theoretical and clinical feuds, without bridges or attempts of any kind at communication. Such relatively independent parties would start to behave within the basic assumption of fight or flight described by Bion (1961).

The second possible scenario would be the definitive victory of biological psychiatry, which would be just another medical specialty, equal to the others, exclusively linked to its neuroscientific basis, bringing neuropsychiatry back to life. Psychotherapists or psychoanalysts, or those who are connected to social approaches, would migrate to other, more agreeable and hospitable climates. For any kind of survival in a world so constituted, the submission to the New Order would be necessary, in a model that resembles the basic assumption of dependency described by Bion (1961).

A third scenario would consist in the maintenance of a large general specialty, mental health or psychiatry, psychology, nursing, *etc.* without qualifiers, like a large umbrella, able to shelter different trends and propitiate the development of specialties, while stimulating dialogue among several of them, and with those having other areas of knowledge.

Obviously I do not need a lot of imagination to figure out these three scenarios; they already exist, and we know exactly where they are. Maybe because I live in a border state, maybe because I have spent so many years going from one field to another in the domains of psychiatry, mental health and psychoanalysis, maybe because I belong to a Department of Psychiatry where this really happens, for all these reasons, I think and hope that the third scenario is possible, because it seems to me to be the one that best serves our patients. Maintaining a space for thinking is the basic proposal of psychoanalysis, and I think that a model constituted like this, in the form of a work group (Bion, 1961), opens possibilities for stimulating integration, reducing dissociation and helping in the working out of mourning, through creative answers.

This may or may not happen. But I think our world and our horizons will be poorer if, somewhere in the future, we are no longer able to re-edit meetings as rich in scientific exchanges and dialogues between paradigms as we are beginning to see in Geneva today.

## 3. SUMMARY

Three different scenarios are offered to the mental health field. The first of them would be that of progressive super-specialisation and microspecificities, in such a way that we would have several psychiatries, psychologies, *etc*, linked to different approaches. The second would be the definitive victory of biological psychiatry, which would be just another medical specialty, equal to the others, exclusively linked to its neuroscientific basis. The third would be the maintenance of a large general specialty, psychiatry or mental health without qualifiers, like a large umbrella able to shelter different trends and propitiate the development of specialties while stimulating dialogue among several of them.

The author pleads for the third scenario and contends that psychoanalysis opens possibilities for stimulating integration, reducing dissociation.

**References**

Agid O, Shapira B, Zislin J, Ritsner M, Hanim B, Murad H *et al.* Environment and vulnerability to major psychiatric illness: a case control study of early parental loss in major depression, bipolar disorder and schisophrenia. *Mol Psyhiatry* 1999;**4**:163-172.

Ahumada, J. (1997). Crise da cultura e crise da psicanálise. *Rer. Psicanál.* Porto Alegre, **4**: 51-96.

Arditi, B. (1988 ) La posmodernidad como coreografia de la complejidad. XVIII Congreso Latinoamericano de Sociologia, Montevideo.

Baladier, G. (1995). Le présent de la surmodernité. *Sciences Humaines,* **5**: 22-24.

Bion, W.R. (1961). *Experiences in Groups.* New York: Basic Books.

Carlisky, N. and Eskenazi, C. (2000). *Resignación o Desafío: un enfoque transdisciplinario sobre la sociedad actual.* Buenos Aires – México: Grupo Editorial Lumen.

Eizirik, C.L. (1997). Psychoanalysis and Culture: Some Contemporary Challenges. *Int. J. Psycho-Anal* 78: 789-800.

Fonagy, P. *et al.* (2000). An Open Door Review of Outcome Studies. *IPA. http://www.ipa.org.uk.*

Kernberg, O (1989). The temptations of conventionality. *Int. J. Psychoanal.,* **16**: 191-205.

Kernberg, (1998). *Ideology, Conflict and Leadership in Groups and Organizations.* New Haven and London: Yale University Press.

Lasch, C. (1978). *The Culture of Narcissism.* New York: Norton.

Lyotard, J.F. ( 1991) Interview. *Zona Erogena.*

Nemeroff CB. (1999). Mol Psychiatry. **4:**106-108.

Roth, M. (1998). *Freud: Conflict and Culture.* New York: Alfred Knopf.

Stolkiner, A (1988). Practicas en salud mental. *Invest. Educ. Enferm.*, **6**(1): 31-61.

Van Der Leeuw, P. J. (1980). 'Modern times' and the psychoanalyst today. *Int. J. Psychoanal.,* **7**: 137-145.

# Scope and Limitations of Psychoanalysis in Clinical Psychiatry

José Guimón
*Professor of Psychiatry; Swiss Psychoanalytical Society*

Psychoanalysis, as a science and as an exceptional instrument for self-knowledge, will continue to grow through its institutes and associations. However, its role in clinical psychiatry has diminished. Spectacular advances in biological research, the presence of psychiatrists in the new short-stay units in general hospitals, and the difficulty of proving the efficacy of community approaches have led to a remedicalisation of the psychiatric profession.

The author believes that the only way for psychoanalysis to play a relevant role in the future of public mental health might be through a somewhat decaffeinated "dynamic psychiatry". This article discusses the scope of this kind of practice, gives data on its extent and indications and comments on the changes needed in psychiatric education.

## 1. THE SCOPE OF DYNAMIC PSYCHIATRY

A report sponsored by the IPA (Fonagy «An Open Door Review», 1999) reviews 50 main research projects (some of them involving a variety of evaluation studies) and makes clear the value of psychoanalysis for many persons with mental suffering. However the authors underline that even if «classical psychoanalysis» remains a set of defined technical operations different from those expected under «psychoanalytic psychotherapy», in practice, the conceptual and process differences between psychoanalysis and the various forms of psychoanalytic psychotherapy have become ambiguous. Furthermore, the psychoanalytic technique varies considerably between analysts, even those trained in the same institution.

In any case, many psychiatrists in Western countries continue to be interested in the so called “dynamic psychiatry”, based in the psychodynamic model. In order for psychiatry to be considered "dynamic", it should at least acknowledge the importance of the unconscious and of transference. Moreover, dynamic psychiatry is traditionally linked with the concept of "conflict" arising between wishes and defences, between different parts of the personality and between impulses and external reality. It also takes into account concepts such as psychic determinism, deficits in intrapsychic structures or internal object relationships. Dynamic psychiatry focuses on fantasies, dreams, fears, hopes, impulses, wishes, and self-image rather than, as is the case in most other approaches, on the careful description of observable behaviour.

Although there is a lack of empirical data, the psychiatrist’s commitment with dynamic psychiatry appears to vary in intensity from one country to another. Surveys have been made in North America, Britain, Switzerland and Spain (Guimón, Fischer, Zbinden, and Goerg, 1998). Data we gathered in the two latter countries illustrate two opposite trends in the adhesion of psychiatrists to the psychodynamic model. For example, although the majority of Spanish psychiatrists (Guimón, 1990), consider themselves well or very well informed about psychoanalysis, only a minority practice psychodynamic psychotherapy (28%) or psychoanalysis (9.1%). In contrast, the profile of Swiss psychiatrists' practices which emerges from our surveys (Guimón *et al.*, 1998) is characterised by a marked predominance of psychotherapeutic activities: more than 80% use psychoanalysis-inspired psychotherapies (Table 1) and one-quarter of them mention psychoanalysis.

*Table 1.* Activities at the individual level in percentages (several answers possible)

| | Switzerland | Spain |
|---|---|---|
| Analytically inspired psychotherapy | 81.3 % | 28.2 |
| Psychoanalysis | 25.8 % | 9.1 |
| Short or focal psychotherapy | 69.2% | 18.2 |
| Relaxation | 42.6% | 49.0 |
| Hypnosis | 17.7 % | |
| Behavioural therapies | 34.3 % | |
| Cognitive therapies | 35.4% | |
| Systemic therapies | 46.8 % | |
| Deconditioning | 35.9 % | 33.0 |
| Psychotherapy + medication | 91.2% | 71.2 |
| Principally medication | 68.1 % | 27.3 |

At the group level, the analytical approach is mentioned by one-third and systemic therapy by almost half of psychiatrists (Table 2). At the individual level, on the other hand, 28.2% of Spanish psychiatrists use analytically oriented psychotherapy, only 9.1% of them do psychoanalysis and 18.2 % mention short psychotherapies.

*Table 2.* Activities at the couple, family and group level B in percentages (several answers possible)

| | Switzerland | Spain |
|---|---|---|
| Family, couple interviews | 79.7 % | 43.9 |
| Family, couple analytic psychotherapy | 38.8 % | 15.2 |
| Family, couple systemic therapy | 47.2 % | 14.1 |
| Analytic group therapy | 14.8 % | 20.2 |
| Other group therapies | 17.4 % | 12.1 |

However, in Spain as in other Western countries, psychiatrists try to maintain an eclectic attitude, using, elements from any of the models of practice, to a greater or lesser extent. In fact, a predominant characteristic resides in the fact that almost all psychiatrists (91.2 % in Switzerland) prescribe medication in association with psychotherapy. This important issue will be referred to later in this article.

A psychiatrist's degree of information on theoretical issues runs in parallel with his/her explicit theoretical approach and with the kind of practice (Table 3). Thus, although most Swiss psychiatrists have fairly good information on psychoanalysis, those who declare themselves «psychoanalysts» appear to be the most selective, by concentrating their reading principally on their specific field. In effect, almost half of them (47.8%) regularly read psychiatric and psychotherapeutic periodicals; one-third of them (38.7 %) read psychoanalysis journals; 16.3 % periodicals regarding family therapy and 12.0 % child and adolescent psychiatric and psychotherapeutic periodicals. The comparison of information levels about the different theoretical orientations between Swiss and Spanish psychiatrists in a way reflects the differences in practices we noted. The latter are appreciably better informed in biology, group psychotherapy and in phenomenology.

*Table 3.* Average scores of the informational level in relation to psychotherapeutic practices

| | Psychotherapeutic practices | | | | | |
|---|---|---|---|---|---|---|
| Informational level (average scores) | Behaviour cognitive | Systemic | Mixed | Short | Analytic. Psycho-therapy | Psycho-analysis |
| Neuropsychology | 2.02 | 1.87 | 1.83 | 1.85 | 1.78 | 1.71 |
| Biological psychiatry | 2.44 | 2.28 | 2.18 | 2.21 | 2.11 | 1.92 |
| Behavioural psychiatry | 2.11 | 1.88 | 1.74 | 1.77 | 1.68 | 1.50 |
| Systemic psychiatry | 2.48 | 2.88 | 2.28 | 2.36 | 2.17 | 1.86 |
| Social psychiatry | 2.69 | 2.71 | 2.54 | 2.58 | 2.49 | 2.35 |
| Family psychiatry | 2.62 | 2.97 | 2.43 | 2.49 | 2.35 | 2.15 |
| Group psychotherapy | 1.91 | 1.88 | 1.87 | 1.94 | 1.90 | 2.08 |
| Psychoanalysis | 2.48 | 2.56 | 2.79 | 2.82 | 2.98 | 3.54 |

The theoretical orientation of psychiatrists depends to a large extent on the kind of training they receive during residency and the type of practice they undertake. Dietz carried out a sociological study on the kind of treatments psychiatrists applied. Those psychiatrists using ECT had received less psychoanalytic training, treated patients at a lower socio-economic status, used more drugs and less intensive psychotherapy. In Spain, we found a link between where psychiatrists worked and the theoretical model they subscribed to. The medical model is backed principally by psychiatrists working in hospitals and those working in centres for alcoholism and drug addiction. On the other hand, those working in community mental health centres are inclined towards the psychodynamic model. All this is, of course, of the utmost importance for the training of future psychiatrists and even for the education of generalists.

## 2. PSYCHODYNAMIC DIAGNOSIS

Patients asking for psychoanalysis still couch their complaints (as do the referring professionals) in terms of traditional nosology. Analysts usually only make use of psychiatric classification to decide whether or not a particular patient should be analysed (*e.g.* a patient diagnosed as having dementia would be rejected); or to predict outcome (*e.g.* the prognosis of phobic symptoms is considered different according to whether the 'diagnosis' is of an anxiety disorder or schizophrenia). As a consequence, psychoanalysts tend to ignore recent research into psychiatric diagnosis and classification.

Freud's concept of diagnosis was closely related to his notion of 'analysability'(Widlocher, 1984). He thus spoke, as is well known, of the 'psychoneuroses' on the one hand, which could be analysed and of 'actual neuroses', 'traumatic neuroses', and 'narcissistic neuroses' which, on the other, could not. Kart Abraham offered a classification of mental illnesses based on the states of libidinal development, and Melanie Klein used a similar principle. Although useful for clinical psychoanalytical work, these classificatory exercises were not based on empirical research.

Current psychiatric classifications (such as DSM-III and IV) have modified the realm of neurosis and character disorders, which have been replaced by headings such as anxiety, dissociative, somatoform, personality, psychosexual, factitious, impulse control, and adjustment disorders. This approach obscures the psychoanalytical understanding of these disorders. If empirically confirmed, Kernberg's (Kernberg, 1980) 'structural' approach to diagnosis could allow the reintroduction of psychodynamic factors into recent classifications. As is well known, he differentiates between neuroses, psychoses, and borderline states on the basis of three main structural characteristics: degree of integration of identity, level of defensive operations, and capacity for reality testing.

On the other hand, as Widlocher (Widlocher, 1984) has pointed out, psychoanalytic psychopathology includes categories such as *manifest* and *latent* content, *secondary* and *primary* processes of thought, *regression*, *transference*, and *mechanisms of defence* and also makes use of categories such as *negative therapeutic reaction* to evaluate change and resistance to change. Unfortunately, psychoanalysts have shown little enthusiasm to systematise these constructs, and when this is attempted, descriptions tend to be based on arcane observational systems and terminologies which place them beyond the use of the average psychiatric practitioner.

A diagnosis in dynamic psychiatry is particularly concerned with factors such as the *strengths* and *weaknesses of the ego*, the nature of unconscious conflicts and defence mechanisms and the structure of the superego. Under the influence of the British school, the importance of the assessment of family relationships, transferential patterns and the so-called *internal object relations* have been taken into account. These components have been appropriately approached through the development of increasingly sophisticated instruments such as Bellak's EFA which was, however, too complicated to be used widely. Recently, the KAPP has allowed for easier utilisation with higher interrater and test-retest reliability. On the other hand, new propositions have been made by a group of the IPA working on the empirical formulation and evaluation of psychoanalysis (Fonagy *et al.*, 1999).

# 3. THE INDICATIONS OF A PSYCHODYNAMIC APPROACH IN CLINICAL PRACTICE

## 3.1. Some Limitations

Psychoanalysis detects disturbances different to those acknowledged by the patient. Frequently, in trying to cure these disturbances, painful consequences can result in the life of the patient. The analyst, moreover, usually works according to some project in relation to what and how the patient should ideally be in the future. This project is conditioned culturally and often does not coincide with the patient's own personal ideal. Sometimes, the paradoxical situation is arrived at, where the patient has to face unexpected problems and live up to an ideal image that, in principle, he or she does not share. The patient's acceptance of the new framing of his or her difficulties and of the new image requires a good deal of indoctrination. This inevitable ambiguity constitutes one of the most poignant ethical questions confronting the psychoanalyst.

Moreover, it is evident that even our usually compliant patients have learned (as happens in every field) to become very demanding consumers of psychotherapy. Psychoanalysis is costly and frustrating. The realisation of its aims can be delayed over long periods of time. The patient seeks immediate results through more agreeable channels. The faith needed to travel along the difficult road with the analyst has been weakened by public controversy concerning the efficacy of psychoanalysis. However, a study of the proposed therapeutic alternatives, shows them to be, for the most part, based on psychoanalysis and to have been unable to demonstrate better results.

## 3.2. The Problem of Indication

The above-mentioned IPA report (Fonagy *et al.*, 1999) demonstrates the value of psychoanalysis through the review of 50 main research projects (some of them involving a variety of evaluation studies). Effectively, psychoanalysis has been shown to be associated with an improvement in the capacity for work and can lead to a reduction in health-care utilisation and in the use of psychotropic medication. Thus, the review concludes that it is cost beneficial and perhaps even cost effective. Estimates of the percentage of patients benefiting clearly and significantly from treatment varies widely across studies from 55 to 96% of patients.

It appears that "completed" and more intensive psychoanalytic treatment tends to be associated with greater benefits than less intensive psychoanalytic psychotherapy, especially for more severe disturbances, although this superiority of psychoanalysis over psychotherapy sometimes only becomes apparent some years after the treatment has ended. In any case, superiority of psychoanalysis over psychotherapy is not maintained at long-term follow-up.

It appears that psychoanalysis may be an effective treatment for severe psychosomatic disorders and borderline symptomatology. Psychiatric symptom scales show bigger changes than personality or relationship scales. Younger children benefit more from psychoanalysis than older ones. On the other hand, however, non-psychoanalytic therapies are better for psychotic patients in terms of improved capacity for adaptation and successful psychoanalytic treatment of severe personality disorder very often requires a combination of supportive and expressive techniques. Behavioural disorders do not respond as well either to psychoanalysis as they do to cognitive behavioural techniques, as do emotional disorders. Furthermore, psychoanalytic therapy at "sub-clinical dose" and of course unduly practiced may have negative outcomes and iatrogenic effects.

In this review it appears that the psychoanalyst's estimate of the therapeutic alliance is more relevant to outcome. Anxiety, guilt and idealisation in the transference may be associated with successful treatment whereas shame, humiliation and existential anxiety are associated with failed treatments.

We could add that many authors suggest that a therapist's function seems essential for the success of any kind of psychotherapy, no matter what its theoretical orientation may be: to provide adequate space for the patient's confiding his or her worries, desires and anguishes to the therapist him- or herself. The therapist thus becomes a container in which all those affections can be processed and, once modified, taken in again by the patient. This "container" meets the patient's needs for emotional contact and cognitive information that lead to passive learning. From that moment, the patient is ready to accept the conceptual framework of the therapist concerning his or her view of the world, of people, of the causes of the patient's disturbances and the means of curing them. At this point, we are dealing with an active learning process in which there is an attempt at modifying the patient's perceptions, feelings, cognitions and behaviour. All the above involve psychoanalytical implications but also existential, philosophic and educational connotations.

# 4. DYNAMIC PHARMACOTHERAPY

## 4.1. Combined Psychotherapy-Pharmacotherapy

### 4.1.1. The Extent of the Practice

The combined use of medication and psychotherapy is a widespread practice today (Thompson and Brodie, 1981; Guimón, Fischer, Zbinden, and Goerg, 1999; Guimón, 2001). In a survey we carried out in Switzerland (Guimón *et al.*, 1998) we saw that combined treatment was widespread among Swiss psychiatrists and even among those who call themselves psychoanalysts (Table 4).

When asked about the different therapies they used, 94% of Swiss psychiatrists indicated that they practiced combined pharmacological and psychotherapy treatment. Combined treatments thus ranked first among individual therapies, before analytically-inspired psychotherapies (84%), short-term psychotherapy (72%) or pharmacotherapy alone (70%), for example (Figure 1).

When respondents who stated that they used combined treatment frequently or very frequently (68%) were differentiated from those who used it rarely or never (32%), we found that this procedure was mainly carried out in institutional practice and less often by those psychiatrists in private practice who also had activities in other settings. Psychiatrists with a biological practice profile and those adhering to the "eclectic model" were much more liable to use combined treatment than were those with a psychoanalytical one (Guimón *et al.*, 1998; Guimón, 2001).

*Table 4*. Other treatments associated with the four types of individual therapy in percentages

| Associated treatments | Types of individual therapy | | | |
|---|---|---|---|---|
| | Psycho-analysis | Psycho-therapy | Behav. cognitive therapy | Systemic therapy |
| Psychoanalysis | 100.0 | 26.8 | 14.8 | 17.3 |
| Psychotherapy in general | 98.8 | 100.0 | 99.8 | 99.6 |
| Analytical type psychotherapy | 96.5 | 85.4 | 80.9 | 80.8 |
| Short psychotherapy | 69.0 | 72.7 | 84.3 | 79.7 |
| Psychotherapy + medication | 91.9 | 95.8 | 98.9 | 98.1 |
| Relaxation | 36.8 | 44.5 | 57.0 | 47.4 |
| Behavioural & cognitive therapies | 25.2 | 46.7 | 100.0 | 64.7 |
| Behavioural therapy | 18.6 | 35.9 | 76.9 | 53.2 |
| Cognitive therapy | 18.6 | 37.1 | 79.4 | 54.3 |
| Deconditioning | 19.8 | 37.6 | 70.4 | 52.8 |
| Systemic therapy | 31.4 | 48.9 | 67.9 | 100.0 |
| Hypnosis | 11.2 | 18.4 | 25.1 | 24.8 |
| Medicinal treatments | 64.0 | 71.4 | 81.0 | 77.4 |
| Family/couple interview | 74.4 | 83.3 | 90.8 | 93.8 |
| Family/couple analytic treatment | 49.6 | 40.5 | 42.4 | 47.4 |
| Family/couple systemic treatment | 28.3 | 49.4 | 66.6 | 89.3 |
| Analytical group treatment | 22.9 | 15.4 | 18.4 | 17.5 |
| Other reference group | 14.0 | 18.1 | 23.8 | 22.9 |

### 4.1.2. The Different Combinations

Combined treatment is neither a unique nor a simple method of treatment. Even if our survey focused on combined treatment by the same psychiatrist and not on the frequency with which Swiss psychiatrists used other specific forms of combined pharmacotherapy and psychotherapy, the results allow us to conclude that a very great variety of combinations exists.

Pharmacotherapy and individual or group psychotherapy can be carried out by a single psychiatrist, a procedure which is frequently called « combined pharmacological and psychotherapeutic treatment ». But the term 'combined' is also used for the so-called collaborative treatments so these terms will be used here interchangeably. Individual psychotherapy and pharmacotherapy can be implemented by different therapists and, in this case, pharmacotherapy can be assured by a psychiatrist or non-psychiatric physician and psychotherapy can be carried out by a psychiatrist (or a psychotherapist who is not a physician), a procedure which is frequently referred to as «collaborative pharmacological and psychotherapeutic treatment». The same could be said when pharmacology is undertaken in parallel with group psychotherapy. Pharmacotherapy can thus be combined with individual and group psychotherapy, the whole treatment being effected by two or three clinicians, either psychiatrists, non-psychiatric physicians or non-physician psychotherapists.

Finally, in inpatient and half-way conditions, a «multiple treatment setting» is the rule, with a great variety of professionals being involved in different activities. As easily understood, these multiple combinations give rise to different technical problems that should be addressed with particular strategies.

### 4.1.3. Advantages and Disadvantages

It has been repeatedly reported (Luborsky, Crits-Christoph, Mintz, and Auerbach, 1988; Luborsky and Singer, 1976) that combined psychopharmacological and psychotherapeutic treatment is better than one of them alone. Karasu (Karasu, 1982) contends that "drugs have their major manifestations upon symptom formation and affective distress, where psychotherapy more directly influences interpersonal relations and social adjustment". He further proposes that drugs may take effect sooner and be of short-term duration, while psychotherapy results may not become apparent until a later point in time, but last longer. He concludes that drugs may be more efficacious for time-limited and autonomous "state disorders", while psychotherapy would be preferable for long-lasting "trait disorders". He thus proposes a "two-stage treatment strategy" in which medication is given to relieve symptoms and prepare the ground for later psychotherapy, aimed at improving interpersonal relationships, social adjustment, and improvement at work. As Gabbard states (Gabbard, 1990; Gabbard and Gunderson, 1999), there are some important exceptions to this assertion: anxiety and depression are "state" disorders that may respond well to either modality. By contrast, attention-deficit disorder is a "trait" disorder that may respond well to tricyclic antidepressants (Ostow, 1983).

Some authors have argued that medication reduces mental suffering thus diminishing the patient's motivation for continuing psychotherapy. Others point out that the transference would be damaged by the introduction of medication. A review of research on these objections (Karasu, 1982) concluded they were unfounded. In combined treatments special attention should, however, be paid (Docherty and Fiester, 1985; Docherty, Marder, Van Kammen *et al.*, 1977) both to the dynamics of the patient and to his or her CNS response.

In the data of the above-mentioned survey, combined psychotherapy is very frequently carried out by the same clinician, especially by psychiatrists working in public services and those with a biological orientation. This kind of practice has of course the advantage of saving time and concentrating the information emanating from the resulting effects of both treatments in the same clinician.

However, transferential issues arising in psychotherapeutic treatment can produce a negative effect on the pharmacological treatment leading to non-compliance or to negative placebo effects. Furthermore, when the treatment involves psychotic, borderline, substance-abuse or other patients with severe disorders, primitive defence manoeuvres and acting-out frequently burn out the therapist.

An alternative strategy is, in consequence, collaborative treatment among two or three different clinicians (Beitman and Klerman, 1991; Beitman, Chiles, and Carlin, 1984). Among the advantages of this approach, there is a sense of relief for the therapist based on sharing the burden of difficult patients (Balon, 1999). In fact, the triangle is a well-known situation for containing conflict and anxiety as has been shown by couple and family therapists.

Patients, on their side, usually report a greater sense of containment and better tolerate the occasional absences of one of the clinicians. It is, however, well known that transference and counter-transference issues can seriously deteriorate collaborative treatment (Busch and Gould, 1993). A great number of coalitions take place among the three sides of the triangle, with side-taking, competition, envy and jealousy (Kahn, 1991). Problems arise mainly when communication among therapists fails and when each of them wants to be the favourite parent, which leads to therapeutically destructive power struggles. For example, some psychiatrists are accustomed to being the primary therapist and feel narcissistically injured by having to share power, believing that their approach is the superior one. Apart from the type of profession, intergenerational differences can add to the difficulties. In these circumstances, patients can be transformed into narcissistic objects.

## 4.2. Medication Compliance

Even when formal psychotherapy is not part of the treatment, dynamic principles are very useful in prescribing psychotropic agents, especially when facing non-compliance, a major factor in the failure of pharmacotherapy.

Reluctance to take medication can arise as a consequence of negative attitudes resulting from side effects which are, unfortunately, frequent and sometimes very disturbing. However, it has been shown that "negative placebo side effects" are also common, in the form of adverse symptoms that cannot be explained pharmacologically (Gutheil, 1982).

These negative placebo effects derive frequently from characterological resistances in the patients. Van Putten *et al.* (Van Putten, 1974, 1975; Van Putten, Crumpton, and Yale, 1976) showed that an ego-syntonic sense of psychotic grandiosity was the most powerful discriminating factor distinguishing schizophrenic patients who did not comply from those who did. An excessive tendency to deny the illness is the cause of many other patients having strong resistance to pharmacotherapy. Some other patients do not conform with pharmacotherapy due to the existence of secondary gains that make them prefer illness to health. These patients may even "cling to their symptoms" when treated, thus making medication fruitless. Still a few reject medication so as not to admit that they are really mentally ill.

The prescribing of medication by a psychiatrist can activate unconscious parental transferences, that may lead the patient to poor compliance. This is particularly true in the case of the so-called "manipulative help-rejecters". The psychiatrist then frequently insists, in an authoritarian way, thus increasing the patient's opposition. Some may even threaten to discharge the patients from treatment if they do not comply, or induce guilt feelings so that patients obey in order not to offend their doctor.

Some psychiatrists may accept the interruption of the treatment just to show the reluctant patient how ill they will get (Book, 1987). On the contrary, some psychotherapists may fail to prescribe a much-needed medication because they narcissistically fear this would bring into question the efficacy of their technique.

Information is not always enough to improve medication compliance, so a certain number of interventions have been designed (Ciancetta, 1983) . Thus, in a controlled study on the evolution of schizophrenic patients admitted to a day hospital, we were able to show that the patients following a group medication program showed better attitudes, compliance and clinical evolution than a control group, apparently due to the fact that both cognitive and affective elements of prejudice towards medication were approached. (Eguiluz, González Torres, and Guimón, 1999; Guimón, 1995; Guimón, Eguiluz, and Bulbena, 1993).

## 5. PSYCHOANALYSIS IN PSYCHIATRIC INSTITUTIONS

The good results obtained with some patients by long-term psychoanalysis in the treatment of neurotic and personality disorder patients on an outpatient basis has not been paralleled with severe psychotic patients treated on an inpatient basis. However, psychoanalytical thinking and personnel training remain essential tools in institutions both for the maintenance of a therapeutic milieu and for understanding and improving the work of the therapeutic teams.

In effect, in this kind of setting, it is assumed that the staff should play the role of an *alter familia* that would enable the clients to have a «corrective emotional experience». However, various difficulties arise in the team stemming both from real problems and from projective identifications that clients put on the staff members. Therapists feel frequently compelled to act transferentially as if they were moved by the projections of the patients. Tensions arise in the team while its members try to become an adequate continent, a «loving therapeutic team», able to take on the needs of the clients and avoid having to assume the difficulties of the staff members. Post groups and different kinds of supervision in therapeutic communities and in didactic communities (Tsegos, 1995) are of great help in avoiding severe emotional difficulties arising in these professionals.

On the other hand, psychoanalytically-oriented group psychotherapy is a basic therapeutic tool in short-term and long-term hospitalisation units for psychiatric patients. The well-known experiences of therapeutic communities, unduly neglected today, are an example of their efficacy. We have reported our experience with several controlled group programs which (Guimón, 2001) have been at work since 1975 in Bilbao, Barcelona and Geneva for severe psychiatric patients in short-term and long-term in- and outpatient clinics. The results of the establishment of such programs were positive both from a clinical and organisational point of view. A particular ward atmosphere develops (Guimón, Luna, Totorika, Diez, and Puertas, 1983) which differentiates from other units which are run with different approaches.

# 6. IMPLICATIONS FOR PSYCHIATRIC TRAINING

## 6.1. The Role of Dynamic Training

The role of psychoanalysis in the future of psychiatry will depend largely on the training programs, due to the resident's identification with his or her teachers and with their ideology during this period. Certain personality dispositions affecting the way an individual approaches life play an important role in the choice of specialisation in psychiatry. The personality profile of physicians choosing psychiatry is changing and becoming more technically- than humanistically-oriented. If this trend continues, there will be, in the future, a host of competent psychoneuroendocrinologists but a dearth of good psychiatrists.

On the one hand, residents have a great tendency to identify with those who trained them during their internships and to adopt their ideology. It is true that when the future psychiatrist begins his or her training, a large part of the psychiatrist's identity - in which his or her professional definition as a physician plays a not so negligible role - is already in place. However, the prolongation of this period of dependence with regard to trainers maintains the psychiatrist in a sort of prolonged adolescence. In what Erikson calls «psychosocial moratorium», he or she has to question their own identity as a physician, to adapt to this new identity as a psychiatrist. In this process, the cognitive information received and the construction of his or her personality through the contact with masters thanks to a more or less unconscious process of identification, play a fundamental role. Indeed, the therapeutic orientation and the general ideology of the psychiatrist are built in part throughout training and become increasingly similar to those of his or her professors.

The type of activities which take place during training and practice, modify ideology. The human being has a tendency to invent beliefs to justify acts. This tendency would explain the adoption of different ideological attitudes according to the types of activity of the psychiatrist. Thus, it is entirely normal that the usual practice of electroshock in a closed institution doesn't have the same influence on the person who implements it as the use of psychoanalytical therapy in an external consultation.

It is necessary, therefore, to consider that the institutional path and expected activities in the program of training post-graduates is particularly important for the training of the identity of the resident as a psychiatrist. Continuing along the same line of thought, the interest has been emphasised of beginning training with activities similar to those of other physicians, such as for example liaison-psychiatry, and thereafter to put residents in contact with a great number of seriously ill mental patients in a short-stay unit.

## 6.2. The New Programme in Geneva

The Department of Psychiatry is one of the 12 departments of the University Hospitals of Geneva and is the only public psychiatric service in the Canton of Geneva (400,000 inhabitants) offering inpatient and outpatient services. No private facilities exist for psychiatric inpatients but 200 private psychiatrists work in the Canton on an outpatient basis; 100 residents work in the Department. A high proportion of residents are foreigners and do not stay in Geneva when they finish their residency.

### 6.2.1. Educational Objectives

The two separate postgraduate training programs in "Psychiatry and Psychotherapy" for adult and child psychiatrists have been under scrutiny in Switzerland over the past ten years and a new adult psychiatry training program was put into practice in 1996. In order to adapt this program to Geneva's Department of Psychiatry and in recognition of the fact that a knowledge of the psychiatrist's daily practice is essential in the formulation of appropriate training objectives, we made a survey of the psychiatric ideology and clinical practices (Guimón, Fischer, Goerg, and Zbinden, 1997; Guimón *et al.*, 1998).) of Swiss psychiatrists and some of the results are given in Table 1, 2 and 3 of this article.

Swiss psychiatrists appeared to have relatively weak biological training whereas, on the contrary, Switzerland appeared to be one of the countries in the world where psychoanalytically-oriented psychotherapies are most widely used. A large number of correlations were obtained amongst all the variables studied, providing some enlightening insights into ways in which training programs might be improved.

### 6.2.2. A New Postgraduate Programme

A certain number of hospital services are accredited in Switzerland to give full training and others to provide a one-to-two year element of training (psychogeriatrics, substance abuse, *etc.*). One year of research is allowed during this period and another year is spent in a medical service other than that of psychiatry. The psychotherapy component of the program is taught through lectures and supervisions carried out by well-trained extramural psychotherapists. Psychoanalysis used to be the exclusive orientation of psychotherapeutic training.

With modifications of the syllabus, the length of the specialisation program has been transformed from five years into six. The components of the theoretical courses have been standardised with a greater emphasis on the diagnoses and biological therapy issues. The psychotherapy element has been better defined. In fact, after one year of general psychotherapeutic teaching, students have the choice between three main orientations: psychodynamic, cognitive-behavioural and systemic and supervisions have to be made in the field that has been chosen. As regards the application of these modifications in Geneva, the program has been considerably concentrated, for the whole of adult psychiatry, and an emphasis placed on biological issues. Consultant supervisors have been hired in psychotherapy, with an orientation other than that of the psychoanalytical.

Moreover, as well as other forms of continual education, an inter-disciplinary «Group Analytical Training in Blocks» (developed by the author in Bilbao and Barcelona in 1976) has been functioning since 1994 in Geneva. More than 250 professionals have undergone this kind of training in Geneva.

## 7. CONCLUSIONS

The theoretical orientation of psychiatrists has been substantially modified in the last twenty years. If, from the dawn of the 20th Century through to the 70s, dynamic psychiatry prevailed in most Western countries, in the 80s and 90s the advance of the biological model was impressive.

In any case, many psychiatrists in Western countries continue to be interested in the so called "dynamic psychiatry" although their commitment with it appears to vary in intensity from one country to another as shown in the data of the surveys done in Switzerland and Spain.

Although current psychiatric classifications obscures the psychoanalytical understanding of these disorders, new propositions have been made by a group of the IPA working on the empirical formulation and evaluation of psychoanalysis.

Psychoanalytically oriented psychotherapy has shown to be efficient for many psychiatric patients and a particular strategy, "combined Psychotherapy-Pharmacotherapy" is widely used among psychiatrists around the world.

Special attention must be paid to the training of future psychiatrists during residency to the dynamic aspects of their practice.

**References**

Balon, R. (1999). Positive Aspects of Collaborative Treatment. In M. B. Riba and R. Balon (Eds.), *Psychopharmacology and Psychotherapy. A Collaborative Approach*. Washington D.C.: American Psychiatric Press, Inc.

Beitman, B., and Klerman, G. (Eds.). (1991). *Integrating Pharmacotherapy and Psychotherapy*. Washington, DC: American Psychiatric Press.

Beitman, B. B., Chiles, J., and Carlin, A. (1984). The pharmacotherapy-psychotherapy triangles: psychiatrist, nonmedical psychotherapist, and patient. *Journal of Clinical Psychiatry, 45*, 458-459.

Book, H. E. (1987). Some psychodynamics of non-compliance. *Canadian Journal Of Psychiatry. Revue Canadienne De Psychiatrie, 32*, 115-117.

Busch, F. N., and Gould, E. (1993). Treatment by a psychotherapist and a psychopharmacologist: transference and countertransference issues. *Hospital Community Psychiatry, 44*, 772-774.

Ciancetta, M. D. (1983). Individual VS. Group medication review programs for chronic Psychiatry patients. *Dissertation Abstracts, Part. B - 44*, 2.

Docherty, J. P., and Fiester, S. J. (1985). The therapeutic alliance and compliance with psychopharmacology. In R. E. Hales and A. J. Frances (Eds.), *Psychiatry Update* (Vol. 4, pp. 524-546). Washington: APA Annual Review.

Docherty, J. P., Marder, S. R., Van Kammen, D., P, *et al.*, (1977). Psychotherapy and pharmacotherapy: conceptual issues. *American Journal Of Psychiatry, 134*, 529-533.

Eguiluz, I., González Torres, M. A., and Guimón, J. (1999). Psychoeducational Groups in Schizophrenic Patients. In J. Guimón and W. Fischer and N. Sartorius (Eds.), *The Image of Madness. The Public Facing Mental Illness and Psychiatric Treatment*. Basel: Karger.

Gabbard, G. O. (1990). *Psychodynamic Psychiatry in Clinical Practice*. Washington: American Psychiatric Press, Inc.

Gabbard, G. O., and Gunderson, J. C. (1999). Making the case for psychoanalytic therapies in the current psychiatric environment. *Journal of the American Psychoanalytic Association.*

Guimón, J. (1990). *Psiquiatras: De brujos a Burocratas*. Barcelona: Salvat.

Guimón, J. (1995). The use of group programs to improve medication compliance in patients with chronic diseases. *Patient Education Couns, 26*, 189-193.

Guimón, J. (2001). *Introduction à la Psychothérapie de groupe*. Paris: Masson.

Guimón, J., Eguiluz, I., and Bulbena, A. (1993). Group pharmacotherapy in schizophrenics: attitudinal and clinical changes. *European Journal of Psychiatry, 7*(3), 147-154.

Guimón, J., Fischer, W., Goerg, D., and Zbinden, E. (1997). Orientations théoriques des psychiatres suisses. *Annales Medico-Psychologiques, 155*(3), 184-201.

Guimón, J., Fischer, W., Zbinden, E., and Goerg, D. (1999). Use and Misuse of Pharmacological Substances: The Question of Noncompliance. In J. Guimón and N. Sartorius (Eds.), *The Image of Madness. The Public Facing Mental Illness and*

*Psychiatric Treatment* (pp. 143-151). Basel: Karger.

Guimón, J., Fischer, W., Zbinden, E., and Goerge, D. (1998). Therapeutic practice profiles, theoretical models and representations of the psychiatry of Swiss psychiatrists. *Schweizer Archiv fur Neurologie und Psychiatrie, 149*, 41-50.

Guimón, J., Luna, D., Totorika, K., Diez, L., and Puertas, P. (1983). Group Psychotherapy as a basic therapeutic resource in psychiatric community care from the General Hospital. In J. J. L. Ibor and J. M. L. Ibor (Eds.), *General Hospital Psychiatry*. Amsterdam: Excerpta Medica.

Gutheil, T. (1982). The psychology of psychopharmacology. *Bulletin Of The Menninger Clinic, 46*, 321-330.

Kahn, D. A. (1991). Medication consultation and split treatment during psychotherapy. *J Am Acad Psychoanal, 19*, 84-98.

Karasu, T. (1982). Psychotherapy and pharmacotherapy: Towards an integrative model. *American Journal Of Psychiatry, 139*, 1102-1113.

Kernberg, O. F. (1980). Neurosis, psyhoses and the borderline states. In A. M. Kaplan and F. A.M. and J. Sadock (Eds.), *Comprehensive Textbook of Psychiatry*. Baltimore: Williams and Wilkins.

Luborsky, L., Crits-Christoph, P., Mintz, J., and Auerbach, A. (1988). *Who will benefit from psychotherapy? Predicting psychotherapy outcome.* New York: Basic Books.

Luborsky, L., and Singer, B. (1976). Comparative studies of psychotherapies: is it true that "everybody has won and all must have prizes?" In R. Spitzer and D. Klein (Eds.), *Evaluation of Psychological Therapies: Psychotherapies, Behavior Therapies, Drug Therapies, and Their Interactions* (pp. 3-22). Baltimore: Johns Hopkins University Press.

Ostow, M. (1983). Interactions of psychotherapy and pharmacotherapy. *American Journal Of Psychiatry, 140*, 370-371.

Thompson, E., and Brodie, H. (1981). The psychodynamics of drug therapy. *Current Psychiatric Therapies, 20*, 239-251.

Tsegos, I. K. (1995). Further Thoughts on Group-analytic Training. *Group Analysis, 28*(3), 313-326.

Van Putten, T. (1974). Why do schizophrenic patients refuse to take their drugs? *Archives Of General Psychiatry, 31*, 67-72.

Van Putten, T. (1975). Why do patients with maniac-depressive illness stop their lithium? *Comprehensive Psychiatry, 16*, 179-183.

Van Putten, T., Crumpton, E., and Yale, C. (1976). Drug refusal in schizophrenia and the wish to be crazy. *Archives Of General Psychiatry, 33*, 1443-1446.

Widlocher, D. (1984). Le psychanalyste devant les problèmes de classification. *Confrontations Psychiatriques, 24*, 141-157.

# Does Child Psychoanalysis Exist?

Bertrand Cramer
*Professor of Psychiatry; Swiss Psychoanalytical Society*

Imagining a psychoanalytical practice with babies as patients would seem incongruous. Though it goes without saying that the baby is the reference point for psychoanalysis in childhood, or that it serves as a model or even a metaphor. But to propose an application of psychoanalysis to babies seems scandalous. First of all, because the baby cannot reveal his or her internal world through the use of words and «talk therapy» is excluded. Then, because speaking about the baby's unconscious is not evident as it is uncertain whether a repression has been able to take root. In addition, it seems difficult to imagine a symbolic creativity in the infant and to distinguish between what is significant and signified. Can we speak of displacement, of condensation in the infant? Can we see the differentiation between primary and secondary processes?

It is difficult to answer these questions in a preemptory fashion; but we can distinguish between two groups of psychoanalysts. There are those who think that only an adult can undergo a veritable psychoanalytical process, which permits the application of metapsychology in order to understand mental functioning.

This is the position taken by certain psychoanalysts for adults who have a strict vision of the analytical framework and of the phenomenon of transference-countertransference.

There is another group which has strongly endorsed the psychoanalytical study of childhood in the baby itself, either via direct observation, or through treating mothers and babies. Their point of view is born out of the opinion that the life of the mind is there from the start, that the baby is much more complex than originally thought and - especially - that the baby forms a whole with the parents' psyches: which is to say that the baby may carry, assume or act out the inhibitions of its mother, be the receptacle of projections coming from its parents and become a part of the parental unconscious. One of the most fertile ideas which has emerged from joint therapy is that the baby is a component of the parental psyche's arena, that it is a sector of it, that it must be heard. In some ways, the baby is a province annexed by the parental psyche, a postpartum, extra-territorial colony. As such, the baby becomes an extension of the parental psyche and will act as a representation.

Two other remarkable functions can be attributed to the baby:

1. As so well said by our much regretted, late colleague and master, Serge Lebovici, it is the baby who creates the parent; it turns its parents into a father and a mother. Its presence creates a new order of mental functioning in the parents.
2. The baby is a material agent of transgenerational transmission: through its behaviour and the symptoms of its conflicts, it represents the identifications, defences which are transmitted from generation to generation. The example of *The Ego's Visitors* described by Alain de Mijolla illustrates this very well.

What is most revealing - for a psychoanalyst - in mother-baby therapy is the illustration of the extraordinary absorption of fantasies and content from the mother's psyche by the child and, in corollary, the strength of the desire to introject maternal content. The content in question is mainly conflictual and can be detected based on the baby's symptoms and maternal anxiety.

Compromises are brokered because each baby is going to react differently to these parental pressures: the adhesion of some will appear complete; others will accentuate their opposition to maternal projective identifications.

What is interesting for the psychoanalyst is to follow the tracks made by maternal fantasy in the child's psyche, then to observe how the pearl is formed to protect against this foreign body, whether it be trauma, seduction, injunction of the superego or a relational method.

Thus, we can observe how the great psychic categories are transmitted: the relationship between the sexes, proximity and absence, love and hate; all these basic values, these ideologies become the object of shared meanings, which will mould the infant's psyche.

The therapist takes part in the building of the psyche and his or her work consists, from then on, in interpreting the alienating pressure created by parental projections and in revealing the baby's own identity.

This work is based on confronting conflicts, defences and the shapes anxiety takes in the mother. We interpret the need for projection onto the child and we interpret the transference that the mother makes to her baby.

What this approach provides in psychoanalysis is, above all, a syntax for parental projections, a healthy respect for the absorption of transgenerational transmissions and an accrued interest in forms of early internalisation.

# Early Disorders in Young Children: The Psychoanalysis of Future Adults

Francisco Palacio Espasa
*Professor of Child Psychiatry; Swiss Psychoanalytical Society*

Research over the past 30 years on the aptitudes of newborns from an instrumental and, in particular, an interactive point of view, has revealed a new field of infantile psychopathology whose *sequelae* can be encountered throughout childhood, from infancy to adolescence.

It must be pointed out that parents contribute to these early manifestations, in varying degrees according to the case, through what we have termed, with B. Cramer, the different conflicts of parenthood.

Mental disorders in the baby can be classified into four groups by order of severity:

## 1. FUNCTIONAL DISORDERS

Functional disorders (sleep disorders, eating disorders, problems with elimination, *etc.*) are the most common. As an example: almost 50% of all babies display symptoms of sleep disorders during the first two years of life. Eating disorders, which are less common, are also widespread in infants.

Functional disorders are frequently transitory and often occur in the context of a parental conflict of a neurotic nature and result in scenarios where parent and child interact. In sleep disorders, the newborn is often treated by the troubled parent as the ideal, cherished baby the parent would like to have been. At the same time, the parent identifies with the image of the ideal of the over-indulgent parent that he or she would like to have had. In order to connect these two ideals of childhood and parenthood, which the parent feels the need to act out in the relationship with the child, there is a tendency to exclude any form of separation from the child, or any kind of expectation of an obligation on the child's part. The child then begins to cry for the parent, particularly at night, when the separations are longest, resulting in sleep disorders.

Eating disorders in the baby very often arise from narcissistic scenarios of parenthood (Manzano, Palacio Espasa, and Zilkha, 1999). They also result from the parent's neurotic conflicts. This concerns mothers who want to idealise themselves as nurturers, to ward off the threat of seeing an image of themselves as the 'not good enough' mother: negligent, incapable, even unworthy and indifferent, something they might have experienced with their own mother. When, in the midst of vicissitudes in breast-feeding or in getting the baby to eat, it shows a lack of appetite either because of periodic fluctuations or more often because of a simple illness such as a cold, these mothers become anxious. «This baby does not want me» they say, putting into words the feelings of unworthiness that they so apprehend. They then start forcing the child to eat; the child reacts by rejecting the food. If this power struggle continues, an eating disorder can be established.

In general, functional disorders can be easily treated through brief parent-child psychotherapies (Cramer and Palacio Espasa, 1993).

## 2. BEHAVIOURAL DISORDERS

Behavioural disorders in the baby with crying jags, bullying, neediness, temper tantrums and/or aggressivity (self- or heteroaggressivity) originate in :

- Parental conflicts of a neurotic nature and are accompanied by various or multiple functional disorders, forming part of the narcissistic scenarios of parenthood. The parent struggles against feelings of being too demanding, too severe, even too suffocating, pretending to idealise themselves as tolerant and excessively indulgent. These conflicts can be treated through brief parent-baby psychotherapies.
- Other more severe behavioural problems in babies are accompanied by mood disorders.

## 3. MOOD DISORDERS

Mood disorders in infants constitute a pathology which has drawn the attention of clinicians in recent years, in relation to mood disorders in parents and notably maternal depression. These difficulties are not, however, the only causes of mood disorders in babies, which are present in the form of:

- Depression in the infant, which is not always easily recognised, sadness (the symptom of depression par excellence) is rarely obvious in a baby. The baby may instead be apathetic, lacking interest or detached from its mother and people in the entourage, as well as from objects in its surroundings which the baby may not explore. To this are added inhibitions at various levels in its own initiatives and activities.
- States of excitation with hyperactivity, instability, repeated crying, *etc.*, a hypomanic bent, constitute a clinical picture of an early defence against the depressing experiences not only of the baby itself, but of the parents as well.

We find the mildest form of mood disorder in the baby to be the result of parental conflicts of a masochistic nature. This concerns parents who considered that they had been «very difficult» as children themselves, creating a burden for their own parents who had suffered from a sub-depressive disorder and exhibited a complaining nature describing themselves as victims of their «tyrannical, demanding and difficult child». The significant feelings of guilt that these parents feel with regard to their own parents leads them to seek expiation through their own children. These children then very rapidly turn «difficult» and «demanding», reciprocating the parent's own childhood feelings. Parents submit to the tyranny of their children with the same sense of victimisation their parents had.

Sadomasochistic relationships resulting from the baby as absolute tyrant and the parent as victim and subject create, little by little, a lack of self-esteem in the child. Effectively, the parent holds up a mirror to the child who sees the reflection of a difficult, even mean child, which leads him, or her, to limit interaction with the entourage. In these babies, there is a progressive build-up of a tendency to control their initiatives excessively, easily interpreted as aggressive by their parents, and a tendency towards inhibitions and a sombre and apathetic mood of a depressive nature. Behavioural disorders precede, accompany or alternate with these depressive manifestations.

The most severe form of mood disorder in the baby is accompanied by attachment disorders of the baby to its mother. This concerns parents who present a severe parental disorder of a narcissistic nature, which leads to aggressive projections onto their children, composed of very negative images of themselves as the children of their own parents. The feelings of persecution resulting from such projections force parents to seek protection through distancing themselves from their children or rejecting them. The great difference with parents presenting a masochistic disorder is that they have a tendency to view their experience with the child who is «difficult» or even aggressive and to see themselves as victimised, whereas narcissists tend to ignore the child, even rejecting him or her, thus perturbing the infant's bond with its mother. These babies are often described as being «capable of going off with anyone» without the slightest sign of anxiety about strangers, but also without a close and specific link to the mother.

## 4. DEVELOPMENTAL DISORDERS

Developmental disorders in babies are found in the framework of conflicts in narcissistic parenthood which are still more severe than those just described. The negative projections of parents onto the baby awaken in them feelings of persecution so strong that the parent, to protect themselves from such experiences, becomes not only rejecting but sometimes openly hostile. As the negative parent-child, or mother-baby interaction which results from this induces guilt in the parent, they seek to hide behind a tendency towards denial by giving themselves the feeling of being «irreproachable» parents or «non-conflictual». This is in contrast to disorders of varying severity linked to the baby's attachment to its parents as noted by the clinician.

The emotional distance of positive affects between the mother and her baby is translated by a deficit at the level of input from the baby as well as by limitations, of varying degrees of importance, placed on activities with the surrounding world which the child does not explore, or very little. This results in delayed development which is more or less disharmonious in regard to language, to symbolic activity, to cognitive abilities or, in more severe cases, to motor skills.

We, therefore, note two forms of developmental disorder in the baby:

- Mild developmental disorders (Multi-System Development Disorders) are found in the framework of mother-child attachment difficulties and are accompanied by mood disorders in the baby. These have been designated in the French classification (Misès) as «Evolutive Disharmonies» and are included in the list of personality disorders.
- Pervasive developmental disorders which sometimes produce very significant delays, are accompanied by serious disorders in the attachment to the mother and affecting the baby's relations with other people. In these extreme cases, diagnosis may be made of Kanner's autism as well as a whole range of infantile psychotic disharmonies. These very severe mental disorders may be clinically detected at a very early age (during the first months or first year of life), but research that we conducted with our colleagues in Pisa (Maestro, Muratori *et al.*) shows that this is not necessarily the case.

Effectively, almost half of all cases later diagnosed as autism or pervasive developmental disorder are not easily identified during the first year of life and diagnosis is more easily made during the second year, between the 15th and 18th month.

## 5. CONCLUSIONS

In conclusion, we can establish a scale of early symptoms in young children based on functional disorders (sleep, eating, *etc.*), ranging from behavioural and mood disorders, to attachment and developmental disorders whose implications are much more severe. Such a psychopathological crescendo has repercussions at the level of difficulties in therapeutic intervention. In functional and behavioural disorders in the baby, child-parent psychotherapeutics have shown themselves to be very effective, often in the form of brief therapy. In contrast, for mood or developmental disorders, therapeutic care is frequently long term and deals most directly with the psychopathological manifestations in the child.

**References**

Cramer B. and Palacio Espasa F. (1993). La pratique des psychothérapies brèves mères-bébés. *Etudes cliniques et techniques*. Paris: P.U.F., Coll. Le fil rouge.

Manzano J., Palacio Espasa F. and Zilkha N. (1999). Les scénarios narcissiques de la parentalité. *La clinique de la consultation thérapeutique*. Paris: P.U.F., Coll. Le fil rouge.

Misès R. and Jeammet Ph. (1993). Classification française des troubles mentaux de l'enfant. *La Psychiatrie de l'Enfant, Vol. XXXI.*

# The Outcome of Psychoanalysis: The Work of the Anna Freud Centre

Peter Fonagy and Mary Target
*British Psychoanalytical Society*

## 1. EVIDENCE BASED MEDICINE AND ITS JUSTIFICATIONS

### 1.1 Reasons Behind the Insistence on Evidence

Psychoanalysis is a clinical intervention. Its aims and ambitions, at least from the point of view of most patients, are clearly associated with those of other healing arts such as surgery, physiotherapy or osteopathy. Admittedly, this is just one aspect of the psychoanalytic enterprise, but one that is crucial to its standing within most of the cultures where it is practised.

Over the last ten years, all aspects of medicine have come under scrutiny, where increasingly both commissioners and funders of medical intervention, as well as those managing and directing clinical services, have embraced the values of "evidence based medicine" (Sackett, Rosenberg, Gray, Haynes, and Richardson, 1996). Clinical judgement is no longer accepted as sufficient grounds for offering medical treatment. It is now expected that recommendations at the level of national policy, as well as at local health care provider level, will be based upon evidence of effectiveness. What factors account for this change?

### 1.1.1 Ostensible Reasons

Evidence based medicine is founded on an ideal - that decisions about the care of individual patients should involve the "conscientious, explicit and judicious use of current best evidence". Much is claimed in favour of this approach, particularly in North America and Western Europe. The arguments in favour include (i) the more effective use of resources, (ii) improvements in clinician's knowledge, and (iii) better communication with patients (Bastian, 1994). From an ethical point of view, the strongest argument in support of evidence based medicine is that (iv) it allows the best evaluated methods of health care to be identified and enables patients and doctors to make better informed decisions (Guyatt, Sackett, Cook, and the Evidence Based Medicine Working Group, 1994; Hope, 1995). All these are good reasons but all were as relevant to medicine in the past as at the moment. So why the current emphasis?

### 1.1.2 The Political Background

The real driving force behind evidence-based medicine is unlikely to be a genuine concern for the quality of care. The movement appears to be largely driven by financial consideration and the hope that health care organisations can reduce escalating costs by focussing on the most cost effective option given a range of treatments. Governments and health funds find the notion of allocating health resources on the bases of evidence quite attractive. In North America, D.K. Eddy in an important JAMA editorial suggested that healthcare funds should be required to cover interventions only if there was sufficient evidence that they can be expected to produce their intended effects (Eddy, 1996). The Australian Health Minister, Dr Michael Wooldridge, adopted a very similar position stating "[we will] pay only for those operations, drugs and treatments that, according to available evidence, are proved to work" (Downey, 1997).

We believe that it is important to derive evidence for psychoanalytic interventions. We are sceptical, however, about the pressures brought on psychoanalytic clinicians as it seems to us unlikely that, even in the face of overwhelming evidence as to the benefits of this relatively expensive treatment, the resources would be available to provide psychoanalysis for a significant proportion of those who require it. In this context it is important to review the philosophical basis of the search for evidence for psychoanalysis in order to gain perspective on the entire enterprise of outcomes research.

## 1.2 Philosophical Concerns

Evidence based medicine represents a practical example of "consequentionalism". Consequentionalism refers to the proposition that the worth of an action may be assessed by the measurement of its consequences. There are at least three problems with the consequentionalist argument, all of which apply to psychoanalytic outcome research: (a) the difficulty in measuring outcomes; (b) the ownership of outcomes (whose interest should be considered?); (c) and finally that consequentionalism may lead to unethical conclusions. We shall take these in turn.

### 1.2.1 Philosophical Questions Concerning the Measurement of Outcome

The first concern is with the measurement of outcome. It is indisputable that many important outcomes of any medical treatment are unmeasurable. Evidence based medicine claims to provide a simple logical process for reasoning and decision making: (i) systematic scrutiny of the available evidence, (ii) drawing conclusions leading to (iii) a clinical decision as to the appropriateness of a treatment. Within this framework, for any decision to be balanced, all relevant consequences of a treatment must be considered. Unfortunately, in the current state of methods of psychological measurement, many important outcomes can only be very inadequately measured.

Psychoanalysis concerns complex internal states such as the degree of distress or pain experienced by an individual. Often these complex states are reduced to simpler, easily measurable ones such as depression (Beck and al, 1961) anxiety (Spielberger, Gorsuch, and Lushene, 1970) or total symptomatology (Derogatis, 1983). A valid objection to such measures (if used without sophistication) is that they are reified and researchers may conflate the measure with the phenomena they were aimed at quantifying. Thus, the BDI score is not depression and the total symptom distress score of the SCL-90 is not equivalent to mental pain. These measurements do not do justice to the complex cognitive, affective and physiological processes which are implicated by these terms.

Even if better measures were found for some domains of outcomes entailed in psychoanalytic treatment, other aspects of the process, such as an 'ethical life', a 'sense of purpose' or 'social justice', may be inherently unmeasurable. Even more troublesome are key domains that are not even well defined, let alone measurable. One such is the "quality of life".

Attempts have been made to provide a metric for this, yet in the absence of a consensus as to what a reasonable quality of life might entail, it is hard to imagine how measurement is possible.

The philosopher Bernard Williams (1972), in an important book on "Morality" noted that values that can be quantified in economic terms, may require comparison with values which are not quantifiable. His comments may be easily extrapolated to the current situation of psychoanalysis in some countries: "Again and again defenders of such values are faced with the dilemma of either refusing to quantify the value in question, in which case it disappears from the sum altogether, or else of trying to attach some quantity to it, in which case they misrepresent what they are about and also usually lose the argument, since the quantified value is not enough to tip the scale" (p 103). Some outcomes of psychoanalysis may indeed be costed, but these may be some of the least important. The cost saved may not "tip the balance" in favour of psychoanalysis.

### 1.2.2 The Ownership of Outcome

The second common criticism concerns the ownership of outcome: "Whose outcome is the outcome of psychoanalysis, anyway?" It may be in principle impossible to decide between the competing claims of different individuals. For example, a treatment that enhances the quality of life of one person may be deleterious to a spouse or an employer. This is particularly evident in the case of the psychoanalytic treatment of children where the treated child's desired outcome may be in conflict with that of the parent's, or indeed that of the sibling. Ideally, notwithstanding the insurmountable practical problems, all individuals significantly concerned with an analysand should be assessed as part of the outcome study. The research enterprise itself is clinician led. It is the clinician-researcher that decides whose outcome will form the basis of evidence-based practice. Thus all outcome investigations, perhaps particularly that of psychoanalysis, will be arbitrary, and limited by the selection of the individual(s) on whom outcome is measured.

An extension of the arbitrariness problem of outcome ownership concerns the status of client choice as an indication of outcome. It could be argued that the client is in a privileged position relative to the investigator in determining whether the treatment is helpful. Interestingly, when user groups are asked they tend to strongly favour approaches to most mental health problems which are psychologically rather than pharmacologically based, or at least they plead for a greater emphasis on psychological help (Seligman, 1995). When individuals perceive their difficulties arising out of psychosocial causes, they understandably seek redress in the same domain *i.e.* the interpersonal. It is also worth noting that psychodynamic therapy often has greater prima facie acceptability than exposure-based cognitive behaviour therapy (for example with patients with OCD Apter, Bernhout, and Tyano, 1984). Yet the desire of the user, "client satisfaction" is not generally acceptable as an adequate criterion for outcome. By this criterion, many treatments known to be ineffective and even harmful, (*e.g.*, recreational drugs such as nicotine to counteract anxiety) could be selected.

Psychotherapy researchers are particularly conscious of the danger of imposing ethnically rooted cultural biases on what is designated as "needing treatment" and to be a "good outcome" (Bemal, Bonilla, and Bellido, 1995). For instance, the achievement of selfhood through the separation-individuation process is one of the cornerstones of psychotherapeutic interventions. Yet was Christopher Lasch (1 978) correct that the emphasis on individual achievement in Western culture is excessive and that an appropriate submission to the goals of the family and community (Kagan, 1984) may be a far better indicator of healthy adaptation? Such differences are particularly acute in the area of child development and parenting. Rogler (1989) outlined some of the practical steps which culturally sensitive outcome research requires. In particular, it is important to ensure that interventions are consonant with the subjective culture of the ethnic group to which it is applied and that instruments used are able to integrate cultural meanings with the pertinent scientific categories. In reality, this is an ideal to strive for, in practice it is rarely achieved.

### 1.2.3 Ethical Concerns

Finally, it is commonly asserted that a uniquely evidence based treatment approach can lead to activities which are at odds with common morality. A good example of this is the success of aversive conditioning and other punishment based techniques in behavioural control of individuals with so-called "challenging behaviour". The fact that there is evidence supporting the efficiency of these techniques cannot and does not make them right.

More generally, ethical concerns arise out of the implementation of randomised control trials. While such trials have the potential to prevent the propagation of worthless treatments, for example insulin coma therapy, they raise major ethical issues in the context of subject selection, consent, randomisation and the continuing care of subjects once trials are complete. Randomised control trials require the clinician to act simultaneously as physician and research scientist. Patients are simultaneously invalids and research subjects. It is questionable if the physicians' moral responsibilities towards patients can be consistent with the recommendation that the patient should participate in a randomised control trial, principally because of this conflict of interest (Hellman and Hellman, 1991).

It has been suggested that such trials may be recommended by the physician if clinicians are in a state of "therapeutic equipoise", that is they are genuinely in doubt about the value of the interventions under scrutiny (Lilford and Jackson, 1995). Such equipoise may be achieved in the case of treatments with moderate effects which might otherwise be obscured by bias and random effects. However, equipoise may not be achievable when interventions have great benefits and risks and then alternative clinical procedures must be evaluated by other methods.

Is therapeutic equipoise applicable to the recommendation of psychoanalytic treatment? Interestingly, neither psychoanalysts nor the opponents of psychoanalytic treatment believe that this is the case. Psychoanalytic clinicians are so firmly convinced of the appropriateness of 4 or 5 times a week treatment that they tend to consider it unethical to recommend less intensive alternatives. Sceptics, on the other hand, feel that the sacrifice demanded of the patient and his/her family is such that randomisation to a psychoanalytic arm is normally ethically unacceptable. In principle, the existence of these opposing views might somehow be combined to construct an attitude of therapeutic equipoise, but in reality it is simply tantamount to what may be an insurmountable obstacle facing a randomised controlled trial of psychoanalysis.

## 1.3 The Need for Persistence

Many other concerns could be raised about the appropriateness of subjecting psychoanalysis to outcome evaluation. We raise some concerns here in part to demonstrate our awareness of the issues and in part to underscore that the clamour for evidence should be met with caution and sophistication. It needs to be recognised that objections to research will not win the day. It is unlikely that the prevailing view, which places controlled studies at the top of the hierarchy of evidence, will change no matter what the strength of opposing arguments. The complexities of issues surrounding resource allocation, the drive to seek certainty and simplicity at the level of policy making are such that alternative formulations will not be heard.

Psychoanalysis is not alone among medical treatments with a weak evidence base. Evidence, to the standards required, is available for relatively few medical interventions (Kerridge, Lowe, and Henry, 1998). The drive for an evidence base for the selection of treatment interventions will inevitably mean a biased allocation of resources to those treatments for which rigorous evidence of effectiveness is relatively easily collected or where funds are independently available to carry out more lengthy and complex effectiveness research. Brief therapy benefits from the former, pharmacotherapy from the latter. Psychoanalysis is further disadvantaged by opposition to many of its fundamental propositions from fellow mental health professionals and influential cultural figures. It is these considerations that drive us to override our concerns with epistemological problems and accept the imperfect solution of outcome research with the overriding objective of preserving the discipline.

The best strategy available to us is to collect all the data available rather than enter an epistemological debate amongst ourselves. The debate is inaudible to those outside the discipline. Further it would sap our energies when this is required for a collaborative effort to make the best case possible for psychoanalysis as a clinical method. Even those of us who are engaged in collecting evidence for the effectiveness of this discipline have major methodological as well as epistemological concerns. These should not be set aside, forgotten about, but nor should they become an alternative focus.

It should be remembered that the debate over the effectiveness of psychoanalysis is one of pragmatics not of principles. There is a clear danger that the therapy that is "without substantial evidence" will be thought by all to be "without substantial value" (Evidence Based Care Resource Group, 1994). Once this idea is allowed to flourish, a cultural change becomes inevitable, a change which at least temporarily has the power to stop the development of our discipline - through the rejection of psychoanalysis as the therapeutic choice, through discouraging young people from entering the profession and through bringing psychoanalytic contributions to mental health disciplines and other subjects into disrepute.

In this chapter 1 would like to review for you our work over the past 10 years on the outcome of psychoanalytic treatment. I am familiar with the impressive work of Professor von Rad and his team and some of our efforts may seem trifling by comparison. Clearly no single centre has the capacity to perform the studies required and only through collaboration between departments and countries will we be able to meet the demand for evidence which faces our field. We are involved in six studies and 1 can provide at least preliminary data on five of these. The implications of these studies, notwithstanding the preliminary nature of the data, are, 1 believe, far reaching both from a clinical and an organisational standpoint. Thus, without further ado, let me start on the first study of diabetic children which George Moran and I completed some years ago.

# 2. THE ANNA FREUD CENTRE STUDIES

## 2.1 The Work on Juvenile-Onset Insulin Dependent Diabetes

This series of studies aimed to establish the relevance of psychoanalytic psychotherapy for children and adolescents with insulin dependent diabetes mellitus who had chronic and pervasive difficulties in maintaining diabetic control. (Fonagy and Moran, 1991; Moran, Fonagy, Kurtz, Bolton, and Brook, 1991; Moran and Fonagy, 1987)

### 2.1.1 Methods

**Sample**

22 children and adolescents hospitalised for poorly controlled diabetes, mostly with episodes of hyperglycaemia, were allocated to one of two clinical units on the basis of their home address. The patients were offered comparable medical interventions and were well-matched on demographic and clinical variables.

**Treatment**

Patients assigned to one of the two units were offered psychoanalytic psychotherapy three to four times per week for relatively brief periods, initially on an inpatient basis. The therapy was carried out by experienced qualified clinicians working with an Anna Freudian orientation. The focus of the therapy was explicitly the patient's developmental emotional conflicts rather than specific conflicts over the diabetes and its management.

**Measures**

Therapeutic outcome was assessed in terms of hospitalisations, levels of diabetic control (HbA1c) and growth.

### 2.1.2 Results

There were clinically significant improvements in diabetic control in the psychoanalytically treated group. HbAlc levels were significantly lower at termination in the experimental group and these improvements were maintained on follow-up. By contrast, improvements observed in the group who benefited only from medical intervention, tended to dissipate by 3 months after discharge. All but one of the psychotherapeutically treated patients showed clinically significant changes but only three of the 11 in the comparison group. There was also a reduction in hospitalisation during the follow-up period in the psychoanalytically treated group.

Two spin-off studies were also reported. Moran and Fonagy (1987) reported that changes in metabolic control were closely associated in time with the analytic material as reported by the therapist. In general the emergence of manifest anxiety in the session associated with psychic conflict preceded improvements in diabetic control by about two weeks.

The second study reported (in Fonagy and Moran, 1991), was a small series of three experimental single case studies. The original sample included three children (one girl and two boys) with significant growth retardation (height below the 5th percentile for age). Growth rate was carefully monitored for all these children. After a randomly determined time period the children entered psychoanalytic psychotherapy. Improvements in growth rate were observed in all three cases associated with the commencement of therapy, although these were more marked in children who were younger at the time of undertaking psychotherapeutic treatment. In the case of one boy an increase of over 10 cm was observed in the predicted adult height.

**Evaluation**

This promising series of studies suffers from an absence of replication, absence of placebo control, small sample size, unmatched length of hospitalisation and the absence of psychological measures of treatment outcome (although measures used were non-reactive). The importance of the studies is enhanced by the known long-term complications associated with this condition and the relatively poor outcome associated with other treatment methods.

## 2.2 The Anna Freud Centre Studies: 2. Chart Review of 765 Cases Treated with Psychoanalysis or Psychotherapy

This was a study of the carefully maintained case records of the Anna Freud Centre, a centre for the psychoanalytic and psychotherapeutic treatment of children under the direction of Anna Freud from 1952 until her death. Case records of the Centre are unusually detailed and to a large extent standardised following Anna Freud's diagnostic profile (Freud, 1962) and incorporating the Hampstead Index (Sandler, 1962). The charts were reviewed by independent researchers and careful attention was paid to achieving reasonable reliability in judgements. (Fonagy and Target, 1994; 1996; Target and Fonagy, 1994a; 1994b)

### 2.2.1 Method

**Sample**

The 763 cases reviewed represented over 90% of the cases seen at the centre for treatment. Some files were not available for research for reasons of confidentiality. Less than 5% of the files were incomplete. The sample was somewhat unrepresentative of the child and adolescent psychiatric population with an over-representation of middle class professional families. Children ranged from 3 to 18 years of age at the start of treatment.

**Treatment**

The average treatment lasted about two years. Over 70% of the treatments were 4 or 5 times weekly psychoanalysis, the remainder once or twice weekly psychotherapy. The treatment orientation was strongly Anna Freudian embracing classical psychoanalytical treatment for neurotic disturbance on the one hand and a somewhat more directive supportive treatment intervention, labelled developmental help, for more severe pathologies on the other.

**Measures**

The key outcome measure was a health-sickness measure - the CGAS score (Shaffer *et al.*, 1983) - manualised for increased reliability as the Hampstead Child Adaptation Measure (Target and Fonagy, 1992). The reliability of psychiatric diagnosis (DSM-III-R) at initial assessment was established with independent raters. A large number of other variables pertaining to clinical presentation, treatment process and outcome were coded. Clinically significant improvement was established using the criteria suggested by Jacobson and Truax (Jacobson and Revenstorf, 1988).

### 2.2.2 Results

Of the emotionally disordered children treated for at least 6 months, 72% showed reliable, clinically significant improvements in adaptation and only 24% had diagnosable disorders at termination. Phobic disorders were most likely to change and depressive disorders least likely. Phobias, anxiety disorders and over-anxious disorders were resolved in over 85% of cases but OCD was more resistant, remaining at a diagnosable level in 30% of cases. Depressed children were least likely to remit. Frequency of treatment and the length of the treatment were both independently positively related to good outcome. High frequency treatments, however, appeared to selectively advantage children with more severe disturbance (multiple psychiatric diagnoses, atypical personality development and pervasive impairments in adaptation affecting social, cognitive and emotional function). These individuals uniquely benefit from intensive therapy. Negative outcomes were most common when non-intensive treatment was offered to this group. Children with disruptive disorders fared less well than those with emotional disorders matched for demographic characteristics and initial degree of disturbance. A large proportion of these children terminated early (33%) but were more likely to do so in psychotherapy than in psychoanalysis. If children remained in treatment, 70% of them were likely to improve to a level where they could no longer be diagnosed. Co-morbid anxiety disorder was associated with an increased likelihood of improvement, as was more intensive and longer-term treatment.

When children were matched for demographic features, severity of disturbance and broad diagnostic grouping and contrasted across three age groups, it appeared that children who were 6 and younger or between 6 and 12 benefited relatively more from psychoanalytic than from psychotherapeutic treatment. Those over 12, however, appeared to benefit as much from non-intensive as intensive treatment. On the whole, younger children showed far larger treatment effects than older ones.

**Evaluation**

This was an uncontrolled retrospective study and the authors were careful in highlighting the weaknesses and limitations of their approach, in particular the biased sample, the lack of manualisation and the relatively primitive standardisation of data acquisition, making it difficult to draw generalisable conclusions. Nonetheless, given the scarcity of data concerning the effectiveness of psychoanalytically oriented psychotherapy and psychoanalysis, the Anna Fred Centre retrospective studies are important both in terms of identifying the limitations of the psychoanalytic approach with children (autistic and conduct disordered children) and also in terms of identifying the patient group for whom psychoanalysis may be uniquely effective (multi-problem, young, severely dysfunctional children with at least one diagnosis of emotional disorder).

### 2.2.3 Discussion: A Little Bit of Theory

Why should intensive treatment be more effective solely for children with relatively severe disturbance? On the surface this observation runs counter to the traditional wisdom of psychoanalytic clinicians - namely that child analysis is likely to be specifically helpful for individuals with so-called neurotic disturbance. The dichotomy between neurotic versus non-neurotic is generally no longer regarded as helpful.

In 1991 George Moran and I tentatively suggested an alternative heuristic - a distinction between what we called representational and process disturbance (Fonagy, Moran, Edgcumbe, and Kennedy, 1991; Fonagy, Moran, Edgcumbe, Kennedy, and Target, 1993). Whereas the former involves defensive or conflict related distortions of unconscious mental representations, (say, for example, an unconscious representation of women as all-powerful and dangerous) the latter involves a defensive or conflict-related inhibition of a mental function which underpins or generates the representational system. Traumatised children, for example, may opt to inhibit their capacity to think about mental states in others, in order to avoid having to think about the contents of the mind of their abusive caretaker (Fonagy, 1991).

We suggested that while disorders in the former category may be adequately addressed by non-intensive therapy, children whose mental functioning was inadequate in certain respects required a more long-term and more intensive intervention. Change in cases of representational or neurotic disorders consists of the reintegration of split-off unconscious aspects of representation, the recovery of repudiated ideas and the addressing of distortions associated with conflict or defence. By contrast, where underlying the disorder is the inhibition of a mental process, such as the capacity to conceive of mental states, therapy works by engaging these inhibited or dormant mental processes. After all, psychotherapy is an activity which forces the individual to exercise a wide range of mental functions, the psychodynamic therapist constantly challenges the patient to engage in their mental world in new and unusual ways. Within the process model, psychodynamic therapy has aspects akin to a kind of psychic physiotherapy. Anna Freud, in a different context, termed these aspects of therapy "developmental help", to differentiate it from the more classical, insight-oriented, approach which she felt neurotic disorders required.

We suggest that milder disturbances do not require developmental help and therefore do no better in intensive than in non-intensive treatment. Process disturbances, by contrast, necessitate the intense involvement of the mind of the therapist with the mind of the patient and this is probably quite difficult to achieve on a once-weekly basis.

## 2.3 The Anna Freud Centre Studies: 3. The Long-term Follow-up of Children Treated at the Anna Freud Centre

This is an ongoing follow-up study asking the simple question if psychoanalytic treatment in childhood enhances adult functioning. The epidemiological background for this study is provided by the growing recognition that children do not grow out of either emotional or behavioural disorder. The adult outcome may not be overt pathology alone but may manifest as poor planning, inadequate sexual relationships, absence of social support, low self-esteem, the persistence of trauma, insecure attachments and adverse life events. From a psychoanalytic point of view, we would explain this as indicating continuities in the representational system. The question is whether psychoanalytic intervention in childhood functions as a protector?

A fascinating recent study from Professor Sir Michael Rutter and his colleagues reported a 20 year follow-up of over 200 individuals half of whom had childhood disturbance aged 10- 11. Measures of psychosocial functioning included a life events schedule, a measure of the quality of planning, particularly during life transitions, adult personality functioning and adult psychiatric diagnoses. The key finding of the project was that childhood psychiatric disturbance was associated with an increasing frequency of severe negative life events during adulthood. These could not be seen as the consequences of adult psychiatric disorder, or continued contact with the family of origin, nor could they be simply discounted as brought on himself by the individual (*e.g.* divorce may be considered self-induced but loss of employment consequent upon the closing of a factory is hard to conceive of in this way). It is more likely that the psychological sequelae of childhood psychiatric disturbance (such as a handicap in understanding minds) leads these individuals into more than usually risky life situations. This, in turn, increases the probability of encountering negative life events. The question we chose to address in the present study was if therapy in childhood has the capacity to reduce such risks. Clearly, such protective effects would only be expected from interventions which had been relatively successful in childhood.

### 2.3.1 Method

**Sample**

Four groups are being recruited for this study: (a) those who received intensive psychoanalytic treatment; (b) those who received once (or twice) weekly psychotherapy; (c) the siblings of the treated groups (in order to control for the effect of shared family environment) and (d) a matched group whose disorder was untreated in childhood. Our subjects are mostly young adults between 24 and 35 and we have excluded individuals whose diagnosis was too severe to permit evaluation using our instruments.

**Measures**

We are using 3 types of measures. First, and perhaps most central, in-depth interview based objective measures of life-events, transitions and plans, current personality functioning, psychiatric and personality disorder diagnosis. Second, self report measures of symptomatology (SCL-90), physical health (SF-36), IQ (NART), personality (EPQ) *etc.* And third, psychodynamic measures of attachment and internal representations of object relationships which provide relatively reliable data concerning the quality of object relationships, the coherence of object representations, expectations concerning other's behaviour, morality, perspective taking, hostility and mentalising capacity.

### 2.3.2 Preliminary Results

We are still in the middle of the study and any results I report are subject to modification as the sample accumulates. In particular, the difficulties in recruiting untreated subjects makes comparisons premature for this group. We feel somewhat more confident of the comparisons between treated and untreated siblings and between treated subjects who achieved a clinically significant change and those whose therapeutic outcome in childhood was poor.

We found evidence supporting our hypothesis that whilst in childhood the vast majority of treated subjects suffered significant adversity relative to their siblings, in adulthood the siblings were more likely to experience significant life events than the treated subjects. In terms of personality functioning, in the work domain all of our sample with the exception of those whose childhood outcome was poor are doing well. In the love relationship domain, individuals with successfully treated psychiatric disorders in childhood appeared to be doing somewhat better than their siblings or the untreated controls. However, none of those unsuccessfully treated in childhood appears to have an adequate love relationship. In terms of friendships, even those successfully treated appear to be somewhat disadvantaged relative to their siblings.

In terms of attachment security, those children whose outcome was relatively good appear to do as well as their siblings in terms of the likelihood of secure attachment. Those unsuccessfully treated appear to be predominantly preoccupied and entangled, whereas those untreated appear to be predominantly dismissing. In terms of the capacity to mentalise, to reflect on mental states, as predicted, the successfully treated group does somewhat better than all the others, whereas those whose outcome was poor in childhood remain unable to conceive of mental states accurately. In brief, successful childhood treatment does appear to be somewhat of a protective factor, although perhaps less dramatically so than we might have hoped. However, where treatment was unsuccessful, this seems to represent a risk factor, with unsuccessfully treated individuals perhaps even worse off than those whose disorders were untreated. We should bear in mind that the samples are small and further interviews may yield quite different observations.

As part of this study we were able to make a number of other preliminary observations of some interest. For example, we were able to compare the information about childhood gained from these retrospective interviews with the original observations carefully recorded by clinicians under Anna Freud's supervision. It seems that the agreement in recall between case-files and adult recollection was relatively high, particularly for physical abuse and discord in the parental relationship. Ratings also matched case-files in terms of the extent to which childhood experiences were regarded as loving, rejecting, pressuring or involving. Thus we may conclude, with respect to the current controversy concerning the accuracy of childhood memories, that these are broadly reliable.

Is there evidence that the forgetting (repression) of adverse experience is associated with psychopathology or poor personality functioning. Here the answer is a qualified "NO". It seems that individuals who are better functioning remember somewhat less well: their recollections are coherent but slightly idealising. They appear to smooth over or forget reporting adverse experiences noted at the time of their assessment. It seems their memory problems arise less from simple forgetting than the reinterpretation of negative experiences as positive. The question arises, if it is sensible to approach psychological therapy by helping people to remember, when relatively good functioning seems to be associated with the capacity to forget. But this issue would take us too far from our topic.

A further interesting unanticipated observation was that actual trauma remembered clearly in adulthood and claimed never to have been forgotten was nonetheless often not recognised by clinicians working 10-20 years ago. Some of the poor long-term outcome may be associated with therapists interpreting these children's reports as fantasy and these individuals repeating such traumata in later development. Perhaps it is not surprising that such individuals remained preoccupied, entangled in their childhood experiences, with their traumatic experiences unresolved. Their psychiatric functioning is less than optimal and they are unable to adapt to either work or social situations. Although we are not assessing this, one must really wonder about the parenting capacities of these individuals and the likelihood of trans-generational repetitions.

A further observation related long-term outcome to technique. Which therapeutic techniques proved to be effective in the long term? Again speaking broadly, it seems that traumatised borderline children are not substantially helped by interpretations of conflict, Oedipal or pre-Oedipal. More simple therapeutic interventions, focussing on the elaboration of the child's current mental state, either with regard to the therapeutic situation or the child's current life appeared to be far more effective for these childhood problems. Focussing on the child's emotional life, his unformulated but perhaps frightening thoughts and fantasies, appeared to bear the richest therapeutic fruit.

Let us turn away from children and the past and move to evaluation of the psychoanalytic approach with adults.

## 2.4 The Anna Freud Centre Studies: 4. The Comparison of Intensive (5 times weekly) and Non-intensive (once weekly) Treatment of Young Adults

### 2.4.1 Method

This was a prospective study where two groups matched for age, socioeconomic status and DSM diagnosis were sequentially assigned to five-times weekly or once weekly psychoanalytic treatment by experienced psychoanalysts. Assessments were made at 18-month intervals by independent raters. The study is still underway and is likely to be completed in 1999. Sample 30 young adults (aged 18-24) referred to the Anna Freud Centre were sequentially assigned to psychoanalysis or psychotherapy. Diagnostic assessments were made by two experienced psychiatrists using structured interviews (SADS-L and SCID-II). All patients in the study had at least one Axis II diagnosis, with narcissistic and borderline personality disorder being the most common. All patients had at least one Axis I diagnosis (mostly mood disorders). No patient had a diagnosis of psychosis and less than half the sample were on psychotropic medication. A significant number of the patients had histories of violent episodes or self harm. About 20% had previous psychiatric hospitalisations.

**Treatment**

Treatments were delivered by qualified psychoanalysts (all Members of the British Psychoanalytical Society) trained in the Contemporary Freudian tradition, strongly influenced by the work of Joseph and Anne-Marie Sandler. The treatments were strongly transference focused. All analysts participating in the study attended a once-monthly supervision meeting chaired by Anne-Marie Sandler. The supervision concerned both the intensive and the nonintensive cases. Analysts had to provide a full narrative account of one session per month which was circulated to the research group and formed the basis of the group supervision. Analysts also completed a weekly rating scale which was a 500 item checklist where they reported the main themes of the treatment and their interpretive work. There was no tape-recording of sessions. Treatment continued in an open-ended way. average treatment length being 3.5 years.

**Measures**

At entry to the study all patients completed the SCL-90, the Beck depression inventory, the Spielberger State and Trait Anxiety Inventory, the Social Adjustment Scale, the National Adult Reading Test and the Eysenck Personality Questionnaire. They were also administered the Adult Attachment Interview, the SADS-L and the SCID 11. The battery was repeated at 18-month intervals. Patients showing significant improvement on at least three measures were regarded as having improved.

### 2.4.2 Results

The results are in the process of being analysed. The key comparison between the outcome of intensively and non-intensively treated patients awaits the completion of a number of psychotherapy cases. The results so far indicate that analytic treatment is superior in achieving clinically significant symptomatic changes. Preliminary scrutiny of the data indicates that improvers in terms of the psychiatric measures could be differentiated from non-improvers on the basis of aspects of the analytic process, particularly analyst's reports of aggression taken up in the transference and the extent and diversity of emotional reactions reported by patients. Transference in successful treatments is characterised by anxiety, guilt, fear of rejection, idealisation and projected aggression. By contrast, failed treatments are typically associated with shame, humiliation, existential anxiety and a sense of boredom and 'cut-offness' on the part of the analyst. There was a relatively high rate of premature termination and this was more common in the non-intensively treated group. Of great importance was the observation that unsuccessful treatments showed differing trends as the analysis unfolded. For example, in poor outcome treatments, the quality of the analytic material gradually deteriorated, affects decreased in intensity, immature mental functions increased together with primitive transferences, and the use of sexual fantasy to support identity. Sadly, there was evidence for the analyst responding by increased disengagement by, for instance, failing to comment on timekeeping problems and concentrating on extra-analytic issues.

**Evaluation**

This study has a number of major weaknesses including the small sample, nonrandom assignment, lack of tape-recording of therapeutic sessions, lack of manualisation of treatment and unequal treatment lengths. However, it has a number of strengths such as the independent assessment of outcome, the use of standardised instruments and the attempt at integrating process and outcome measures.

## 2.5 The Anna Freud Centre Studies: 5. The Evaluation of a Psychotherapeutic Day Hospital

Anthony Bateman and I undertook to explore how effective an intensive psychodynamic therapy based day hospital programme could be for individuals diagnosed with borderline personality disorder.

### 2.5.1 Method

**Sample**

44 patients were randomised to treatment as usual or the day hospital. All patients in the sample met both DSM-IIIR and Gunderson criteria for borderline personality disorder. The patient group showed severe psychiatric disorders including mood disorders, eating disorders, dysthymia and borderline, narcissistic or paranoid personality disorder. There was a high prevalence of physical abuse, sexual abuse, early loss, rape *etc.*

**Treatment**

The control treatment was variable. Almost three-quarters received day hospital care in non-psychotherapeutic settings. In addition they benefited from day centres, polypharmacy, community support, outpatients services and occasional inpatient services. The experimental group had individual psychotherapy under close supervision, group psychoanalytic psychotherapy, expressive therapy and the staff received consistent support. The theoretical framework included a focus on disorganised attachment manifesting as an intolerance of closeness, addressing gross limitations of mentalising capacity, assistance in developing a transitional state of mind, and a close focus on the counter-transference.

**Measures**

The most important measures were suicidal and self-mutilatory acts, hospitalisation, length of inpatient episodes and self-report measures of symptom distress and mood.

### 2.5.2 Results

There was a dramatic drop in the number of suicide attempts after six months of treatment, maintained over the 18 months of day hospital treatment. There was a somewhat slower reduction in the rate of self-mutilating behaviour which decreased to under 40% in the final 6 months of the trial. The number of hospital admissions during the 18 months of the trial remained low for the day hospital group but was on the increase again for the control group. The more important variable of length of hospitalisation showed a similar patter.

Impressively, depression continued to decline for the day hospital group but was unchanged for the treatment as usual control group. Symptom severity on the SCL-90 also declined sharply. Other self-report measures yielded very similar results.

**Evaluation**

This is the first randomised controlled trial of a psychodynamic treatment for borderline personality disorder. It should be added that a programme such as this has many features beside therapy which may have beneficial effects. We believe that certain key features of the programme account for its powerful effects, at least in the short term. These include its consistency and reliability, its highly structured character, its intensity, its coherence coupled with a flexible treatment approach, its relationship focus and the individualisation of care plans.

## 3. CONCLUSIONS

None of these are uniquely psychoanalytic ideas, yet I believe they exemplify the modern psychodynamic approach. In evaluating our work, we are forced to face up to the fact that none of us any longer practice Freud's therapy. We have learned a great deal from Freud and his great discovery that unconscious feelings and beliefs are critical to understanding both normal and pathological mental states remains a core aspect of our work. Perhaps what we have learned over the past 100 years is that the specific unconscious affects or beliefs, Oedipal conflicts, anal fixations, anaclitic depression and the like are not what makes our work psychoanalytic. The content of interpretation varies from patient to patient, from country to country, from analyst to analyst. The formal structure of psychoanalytic intervention I believe remains the same across these divides and constitutes the essence of what we mean by psychoanalysis. I believe that when we systematically evaluate the effectiveness of one human being elaborating on the non-conscious mental states of another in the context of an intimate personal relationship we are confronted with a psychiatric intervention of remarkable potency.

Our work at the Anna Freud Centre is but a small fragment of what needs to be done, but could be done quickly and effectively, to demonstrate to others the value of our approach. International collaboration will be essential to provide funders with compelling evidence for the value of our clinical intervention. Psychoanalysts have been shy of public exposure, fearing humiliation or worse. While psychoanalysis may not be a panacea, the emerging evidence underscores that we have nothing to be ashamed of and that our theory and technique may well be uniquely helpful in assisting those whose life experience and perhaps constitutional make-up has put them at greatest disadvantage. The reasons for evaluation studies may not be the ones which clinicians desire but doing them will teach us more about our patients, our work and ourselves.

**References**

Apter, A., Bernhout, E., and Tyano, S. (1984). Severe obsessive compulsive disorder in adolescence: A report of eight cases. *Journal of Adolescence*, 7, 349-358.

Bastian, H. (1994). The power of sharing knowledge. Consumer participation in the Cochrane Collaboration. Oxford: UK Cochrane Centre.

Beck, A.T. *et al.*, (1961). An inventory for measuring depression. *Archives of General Psychiat.*

Bernal, G., Bonilla, J., and Bellido, C. (1995). Ecological validity and cultural sensitivity for outcome research: Issues for the cultural adaptation and development of psychosocial treatments with hispanics. *Journal of Abnormal Child Psychology*, 23, 67-82.

Derogatis, L. R. (1983). SCL-90R: Administration, scoring and procedures Manual II. Towson, MD: Clinical Psychometric Research Inc.

Downey, M. (10 May 1997). Trust me I'm a doctor. Sidney Morning Herald, pp. 1.

Eddy, D. K. (1996). Benefit language: criteria that will improve quality while reducing costs. *Journal of the American Medical Association*, 275, 650-657.

Evidence Based Care Resource Group. (1994). Evidence based care 1. Setting priorities: how important is this problem. *Canadian Medical Association Journal*, 150, 1249-1254.

Fonagy, P. (1991). Thinking about thinking: Some clinical and theoretical considerations in the treatment of a borderline patient. *International Journal of Psycho-Analysis*, 72, 1-18.

Fonagy, P., Moran, G., Edgcumbe, R., and Kennedy, H. (199 1). The roles of mental representation and mental process in therapeutic action.

Fonagy, P., and Moran, G. S. (1991). Studies of the efficacy of child psychoanalysis. *Journal of Consulting and Clinical Psychology*, 58, 684-695.

Fonagy, P., Moran, G. S., Edgcumbe, R., Kennedy, H., and Target, M. (1993). The roles of mental representations and mental processes in therapeutic action. The Psychoanalytic Study of the Child, 48, 9-48.

Fonagy, P., and Target, M. (1994). The efficacy of psychoanalysis for children with disruptive disorders. *Journal of the American Academy of Child and Adolescent Psychiatry*, 33, 45-55.

Fonagy, P., and Target, M. (1996). Predictors of outcome in child psychoanalysis: A retrospective study of 763 cases at the Anna Freud Centre. *Journal of the American Psychoanalytic Association*, 44, 27-77.

Freud, A. (1962). Assessment of childhood disturbances. *The Psychoanalytic Study of the Child*, 17, 149-158.

Guyatt, G. H., Sackett, D. L., Cook, D. J., and the Evidence Based Medicine Working Group. (1994). Users' guides to the medical literatures. *Journal of the American Medical Association*, 271, 59-63.

Hellman, S., and Hellman, D. S. (1991). Of mice but not men. Problems of the randomised clinical trial. *New England Journal of Medicine*, 324, 1585-1589.

Hope, T. (1995). Evidence based medicine and ethics. *Journal of Medical Ethics*, 21, 259-260.

Jacobson, N. S., and Revenstorf, D. (1988). Statistics for assessing the clinical significance of psychotherapy techniques: Issues, problems, and new developments. *Behav. Assess*, 10, 133-145.

Kagan, J. (1984). The Nature of the Child. New York: Basic Books.

Kerridge, I., Lowe, M., and Henry, D. (1998). Ethics and evidence based medicine. *British Medical Journal*, 316, 1151-1153.

Lasch, C. (1978). The Culture of Narcissism: American Life in an Age of Diminishing Expectations. New York: Norton.

Lilford, R., and Jackson, J. (1995). Equipoise and the ethics of randomizations. *Journal of Research in Social Medicine*, 88, 552-559.

Moran, G., Fonagy, P., Kurtz, A., Bolton, A., and Brook, C. (199 1). A controlled study of the psychoanalytic treatment of brittle diabetes. *Journal of the American Academy of Child and Adolescent Psychiatry*, 30, 926-935.

Moran, G. S., and Fonagy, P. (1987). Psychoanalysis and diabetic control: A single-case study. *British Journal of Medical Psychology*, 60, 357-372.

Rogler, L. H. (1989). The meaning of culturally sensitive research in mental health. *American Journal of Psychiatry*, 146, 296-303.

Sackett, D. L., Rosenberg, W. M., Gray, J. A. M., Haynes, R. B., and Richardson, W. S. (1996). Evidence based medicine: What is is and what it isn't. *British Medical Journal*, 312, 71-72.

Sandler, J. (1962). The Hampstead Index as an Instrument of Psychoanalytic Research. International Journal of Psycho-Analysis, 43, 287-291.

Seligman, M. E. P. (1995). The effectiveness of psychotherapy. *Am Psychologist*, 50, 965-974.

Shaffer, D., Gould, M. S., Brasie, J., Ambrosini, P., Fisher, P., Bird, H., and Aluwahlia, S. (1983). A children's global assessment scale (CGAS). *Archives of General Psychiatry*, 40, 1228-123 1.

Spielberger, C. D., Gorsuch, R. L., and Lushene, R. E. (1970). The State-Trait Anxiety Inventory (Self-Evaluation Questionnaire). Palo Alto, CA: Consulting Psychologists Press.

Target, M., and Fonagy, P. (1992). Raters' Manual for the Hampstead Child Adaptation Measure (HCAM) .

Target, M., and Fonagy, P. (1994a). The efficacy of psychoanalysis for children with emotional disorders. *Journal of the American Academy of Child and Adolescent Psychiatry*, 33, 361-371.

Target, M., and Fonagy, P. (1994b). The efficacy of psychoanalysis for children: Prediction of outcome in a developmental context. *Journal of the American Academy of Child and Adolescent Psychiatry*, 33, 1134-1144.

Williams, B. (1972). Morality. Cambridge: Cambridge University Press.

# Vestiges of Childhood and Adult Psychoanalysis

Florence Quartier-Frings
*Swiss Psychoanalytical Society*

«Thirty or forty years later...» an adult, who no longer remembers the very young child he or she once was, decides to undergo analysis. The client may be the victim of disturbing elements in his or her life, inexplicable repetitions, agonised suffering... or may not. The client may be a victim of fears that make life uncomfortable or worse, cutting the person off from the immediacy of experience, repressing emotional reactions. All this is linked to the child who once existed, but if so, how?

## 1. THE IMPORTANCE OF THE PAST

The importance accorded by psychoanalysts to the past has been unquestioned: it has worked on the assumption that the past leaves its mark on the present, a hypothesis which has never been disputed. In 1905, Freud said that he had become: «finally more skilled at distinguishing between illusions of memory and the remnants of real events.» This shows how very complex it is, *a priori*, to undertake psychoanalytical investigations of the past. But beyond conventional wisdom on the importance to be accorded to the past, questions arise: what are the signposts to the past and how do we find them? Herein lie the arguments in a debate which has lasted since the beginning of the history of analysis and is among those which have contributed the most – and continue to do so - to the evolution of techniques of interpretation. For example, during the years 1911-1915, Karl Abraham imagined that the past could re-emerge, in an identical form, brought back by the flow of the regressive libido which in some ways carried with it the flotsam of old elements. He spoke often of the auto-eroticism of the neurotic, as a manifestation of a return and/or the persistence of a stage which should have been concluded during development.

The past, in this concept, is always childhood and even more, a shameful childhood, a sign of immaturity, a tendency toward regression, that should be made to disappear. But when Karl Abraham speaks in these terms of the past, he does so from the position of very brief experience. It was a beginning, an attempt to create order, interesting but is obviously insufficient for our uses today.

## 2. AN INCREASINGLY COMPLICATED LINK

We should not be surprised to see the terms of the debate being modified, unless we wish to turn psychoanalysis into a museum artefact. Theory remains subject to practice and its evolution. Thus, it would appear that as practices diversify and become more complicated, the links between the present and the past become increasingly intricate and complex, to a degree that the first psychoanalysts could only imagine.

This is a very complicated debate, the full understanding of which requires a detailed textual study if we are to gain a critical retrospective reading. This reveals an ongoing tension between practice and analytical theory in:

- an attempt to objectively create order out of the past, and
- audacious research, both difficult and risky, to recreate a hypothetical past whose reality is plausible but not verifiable.

Today, this tension forms an integral part of the analytical process. It is within the framework of this exercise and the way it is implemented that the differences between psychoanalysis, psychotherapy and/or one-on-one psychoanalysis will be found in the future.

The analyst bases his or her work on objective knowledge and should not disregard this. Analytical research accumulated over the last decades has revealed an increasingly clear picture of the series of problems occurring in the child and in the adult; and to revert to the theme of this round table, the precise distinctions that have been made between the difficulties arising in the adult, as they are expressed in therapy, and those which affect development during childhood itself. Here in Geneva, there is no need to look far to acquire very clear ideas on the subject: the work pioneered by Bertrand Cramer looked into the birth of the infant, its surroundings, its reactions to confrontation with specific difficulties, joys and hope. It was not always so. Great confusion arose in the work of the first child psychoanalysts, where rapidly formulated analogies were made, based on simple resemblances between adult psychosis and certain expressions of joy or rage in very small children. Other oversimplified analogies led to definitions of the symbiosis of some very complicated behaviours in early childhood but which, in fact, are never found *per se* in the adult, even one who is very disturbed. Here again, while these pioneering efforts remain noteworthy, in terms of the links between a forgotten past and current experience, much of this work dates back to the Fifties and appears partially obsolete to us.

Today, the finer distinctions drawn between problems arising from childhood and those of the adult have very important consequences for the work of interpretation. We know, for example, that it is not necessary to point to an analogy between now and the 'old days', to cause mental transformations in the adult to occur.

## 3. MAKING MEMORIES PERCEPTIBLE

All these elements, viewed objectively, are now well known. Others, emanating from the neurosciences, deal, for example, with memory and the cognitive process. However, these elements do not permit the psychoanalyst to rid him- or herself of the gesture - at the behest of the transferential link - of following that other path to which I have already alluded: the past must be recreated, sometimes starting from scratch, and without even knowing if the blocks out of which it must be built were really present in the childhood of the adult subject.

Herein lies one of the most remarkable points in analytical practice. It is most easily «visible», most easily comprehensible, from the point of view of the transferential link which will, over time, become considerably modified, refined, deepened and complex. This link, belonging to analytical practice, has never ceased to grow in strength or in detail. It has become a veritable tool of investigation: many analysts have become advocates of (and experts in) a particular area of research into the past: on the one hand, they know how to detect the almost imperceptible signs which emerge during a session, directly from the mists of childhood. They, therefore, know how to deepen and sharpen their inquiry. But there is more. Analysts have also learned how to discern the unknown, delineate the unknowable, detecting for example a « black hole » which may provide a gateway directly to the genesis of narcissism: to that place where it was created, amalgamated over time, at the very beginnings of life. Analysts have also become skilled at making memories which elude the conscious mind perceptible. A qualitative concept is added onto the quantitative search previously mentioned. But this consists of tracing details, the insignificant, minutiae: forgotten and re-emerging in an unforeseen and disordered manner. The setting must evoke the atmosphere of childhood, summoning it once again while dealing with current affects, words, complicated memories, that the subject may not even know existed as such.

The influence of the past must then be evaluated on the basis of furtive elements which differ from indirect factors: this can be a way of telling one's own story where the vestiges of childhood are more significant than the story itself. It can be an unconscious means of identifying with certain behaviours of the father (or the mother). Though it remains to be seen whether this identification is related to the figure of the father in childhood, to that of adolescence or even to the father about whom the entourage spoke and who differs, probably, as an entity from the person with whom the small child was directly in contact. Consideration must also be given to dream interpretation which, in the adult, occurs in the course of transferential associations and allows us to discover some frequently, very unexpected aspects of persistent childhood influences.

It must be pointed out that these discordant elements which seem to arise from the past, are of uncertain origin; we cannot find the point at which they were born. In any case, they were transformed over time, but subsist in some form. They may have contributed, directly or, on the contrary, through tortured transformations, to constituting the adult subject's past. In a certain way, these elements of the past, by expressing themselves indirectly, obliterate the adult subject's present life. The adult complains about them, and this complaint must be picked up in analysis. But the past, and the vestiges of childhood it contains, are also a forceful source of enriching experiences.

We can, therefore, see the great interest that exists in debating the idea of the past. Particularly as this theme also carries a link to very current questions on the challenges of working in psychoanalysis, of inquiring into the finality of analysis and how to set markers for future development.

## 4. CONCLUSION

Today, we consider the past to be rich in complexity, impossible to completely elucidate but that it ceaselessly floods into the present, often in a latent manner. There is no point in thinking we must rid ourselves of the past, that it is necessary to dispel the traces of childhood in order to gain access, through analysis, to a maturity which is devoid of the thrilling joy and devastating sadness which are reputed to be the trademarks of immaturity. In adult psychoanalysis, the question is rather that of revealing the signposts of the past, identifying their current impact, diminishing their weight should the need exist, especially when the subject does not realise the burden he or she is carrying. For example, it is important to detect what arises from the genesis of narcissism, what continues to nourish the present or what can - sometimes - be devouring it. Activating (or re-activating) variations in the expression of instinctive currents which - from birth to death - feed the psyche and contribute to the organisation and disorganisation of the subject's outlook. It is also a question of detecting which past influences are persistent and possibly unchangeable, and which are in the process of being transformed, modified, but are still inadequately separated from childhood. Without haste, with constancy and curiosity, the analyst and sometimes simultaneously the subject, discover how much the past can discreetly make itself heard. Of course, it often conceals much pain which may have been partially forgotten. But placing the accent on the role of the past opens a door onto one of the most beautiful panoramas offered by analysis: the possibility that the past is a source of potential dynamism, fed by an inexhaustible energy; a capacity for ceaselessly renewing the work on the past, on our memory and on the paths that are revealed.

# Concluding Remarks

Nicos Nicolaïdis
*Chair, Scientific Committee; Swiss Psychoanalytical Society*

«Challenges in Psychoanalysis in the 21st Century: Psychoanalysis, Health and Psychosexuality in the Era of Virtual Reality» was the theme of this Interregional Conference. Synonymous with virtual reality are potential, dynamics. The journey through the work of Freud is the paradigm of this virtual reality. Basing ourselves on his discovery of infantile sexuality, whose evolutionary point is the Oedipal organisation of genitality, proposing the idea of fantasies and psychic reality, Freud gave an unconscious dimension to Kantian consciousness and to that of phenomenologists at the end of the 19th century.

The famous «meta» of metapsychology does not only signify the aftermath, but also the experience, the depth even the third dimension of the iceberg.

Introducing narcissism and then the second topographical point of view, he showed dialectically that instinct and object, *i.e.* the intrapsychic and the intersubjective are an echo of each other. And the concept of the id, brings us back to the psychic link with biology. We see the same virtual research in the work of his disciples.

The ideas deliberated in these meetings and the discussions they gave rise to, centred around this evolutionary Freudian and post-Freudian axis which has at its epicentre the human dimension, virtual research by Freud: Eros, the libido, elements which, in a positive or negative fashion, characterize the human condition.

Thus, if psychoanalysis is humanism, it will, in spite of all the ills of civilisation which rain down on us, survive from here to eternity.

We must first recognize our debt to Sara Zac de Filc, who inspired and organised the encounter in which this book is based. The distance between Buenos Aires and Geneva was considerably shortened by Mauricio Gitnacht who provided the link. Professor José Guimón, aided by the invaluable assistance of Mary Ritchie, mobilised with efficiency and enthusiasm, the infrastructure of his university service. In collegial, amicable collaboration with the Scientific Committee, he was the architect of the final form of this event, giving proof of the close cooperation that exists between psychiatry and psychoanalysis. We are most grateful to him.

# Index